HONEY, GARLIC, & VINEGAR

home remedies & recipes

Cleaning tips for the kitchen

The next couple of columns will be devoted to the little things that help keep your home clean and sparkling. That will help you in every day life, as well as when you want to sell it.

Today, we'll deal with the kitchen, here's a lot of little cleaning secrets.

To clean up the yellowing that occurs on some appliances, mix together 1/2 cup of bleach, 1/2 cup of baking soda and four cups of warm water. Apply the mixture, let stand for about 10 minutes and then wipe clean and dry.

Instead of commercial waxes, try rubbing the fridge or stove down with rubbing alcohol, or use club soda for quick clean-ups. It cleans and shines at the same time.

To loosen grime which gathers on your can opener, use an old toothbrush and then run a paper towel through the cutting surfaces... presto! It's clean.

For those tarnished copper pots or kettles, fill a spray bottle with vinegar and three tablespoons of salt. Spray it on, let it stand and wipe it off.

The oven is probably the most used and hardest to clean item in your kitchen. Try setting the oven on warm for about 20 minutes and then put a small dish of amonia on the top rack and a pot of boiling water on the bottom and close the oven. Let it sit in there overnight. In the morning, air it out and you can wipe off even hard baked-on grease easily.

To clear a grease-clogged drain, pour in a cup of salt and a cup of baking soda, followed by a kettle of boiling water. It cuts through the grease like magic. And those coffee grounds? Throw them in the trash, not down your sink!

A box of baking soda in the refrigerator, does absorb odors. To make it smell even better, put a little vanilla on a piece of paper towel or cotton ball and leave it in there.

To really clean a white porcelain sink, spread paper towels on the bottom and soak with bleach for an hour or so.

To remove water spots from stainless steel sinks, use rubbing alcohol or white vinegar on a sponge.

And a final "sink trick". Club soda will shine up stainless steel in a jiffy. It's an old bartender's trick!

Try these little tips and your kitchen will be bright and shiny all the time.

HONEY, GARLIC, & VINEGAR

home remedies & recipes

the people's guide to Nature's wonder medicines

by
Patrick Quillin, PhD,RD,CNS

**published by
The Leader Co., Inc.
North Canton, OH**

📖 **Other books by Dr. Patrick Quillin**

La Costa Prescription for Longer Life, Fawcett Crest, NY, 1985
Healing Nutrients, Random House, NY, 1987
La Costa Book of Nutrition, World Almanac, NY, 1988
Safe Eating, Evans, NY, 1990
Adjuvant Nutrition in Cancer Treatment, CTRF, Arlington Hts, IL, 1993
Amish Folk Medicine, Leader Company, N. Canton, OH, 1993
Beating Cancer with Nutrition, Nutrition Times Press, Tulsa, 1994
Wisdom & Healing Power of Whole Foods, Vitamix, Cleveland, 1994
Healing Secrets from the Bible, Nutrition Times Press, Tulsa, 1996

Printed in Canada

Quantity   discounts   are   available   from:
The Leader Company, Inc. 📖
931 N. Main #101
N. Canton, OH 44720
phone 216-494-6988; fax 216-494-6989

On your letterhead, include information concerning the intended use of the books and the number of books you wish to purchase.

CONTENTS

DEDICATION

To my mother, Margaret Mary Quillin, who instilled in me an appreciation of the beauty to be found in Nature. God Bless You.

ACKNOWLEDGEMENTS

For my incredible wife, Noreen, who spent endless hours assisting in this manuscript and for her unconditional love that nourishes my soul.

For the thousands of scientists around the world who have transcended criticism and a lack of funding in their pursuit of the truth regarding the therapeutic value to be found in natural, unpatentable substances.

Chapter 1

📖

NATURE'S PHARMACY CAN HEAL YOU

simple solutions for complex modern health problems

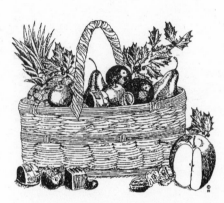

"Nature, to be commanded, must be obeyed." Francis Bacon, 1620 A.D.

❀ PERSONAL PROFILE. FJ was a busy attorney with more money than health. He had already suffered one heart attack and was under constant medical surveillance since he had all the signs of having another heart attack. FJ came to me for help. The medication he was taking was causing impotence and problems concentrating on his work. I suggested that we try a different approach to reversing his heart disease. While continuing with his medication, I put him on a low fat diet, daily exercise, with lots of garlic, vinegar, vitamin E, fish oil, and chromium supplements. Within 8 weeks, FJ's doctor remarked about the changes in his risk factors. Within 12 weeks, FJ was taken off medication and found a newfound passionate romance with his wife and his work. This is just one example of how people can find near-miraculous relief in Nature's pharmacy.

Congratulations on your wise investment in this book!! Nature has the most remarkable, inexpensive, and non-toxic healing agents on the planet earth. Nature's pharmacy has been around much longer than mankind's pharmacies.

While drugs and surgery can only temporarily deal with symptoms, Nature's "pharmacy" can actually prevent and reverse most ailments. Of all the "superfoods" provided in Nature, honey, garlic, and vinegar are perhaps the "dream team" of concentrated healers.

In this unique trio, we have:
• Nature's sweetest food--honey, from her most industrious workers--bees
• Nature's most potent and versatile healing herb, flavorful spice, and nourishing vegetable-- garlic
• Nature's most potent and versatile fermented food--vinegar.

Your body wants to be healthy. But in many Americans, we are not providing the proper "building materials" to allow the body to maintain health. Just like if a home builder is not supplied with the proper array of high quality lumber, concrete, pipes, nails, etc.; then the workers cannot create a strong house. Though humankind certainly has developed some advanced tools, like notebook computers, satellite communication, and laser surgery, we still cannot make a baby, or an apple or even leather. We have to rely on Nature for these gifts. The same goes for our health. Good health does not come from an endless series of trips to the doctor. Good health has to be earned by working hand-in-hand with Nature.

Given the opportunity, your body should provide you with good to excellent health for the better part of 80 to 120 years. If you are not getting this level of performance from your body, then examine your diet, exercise, attitude, and exposure to toxins. These four major components influence how you feel, how often you get sick, how much zest you get out of life, and how long you will live.

✍   Honey, garlic, and vinegar are very special "prescriptions from Nature's pharmacy" to get you on the road to optimal health. Using these foods in the context of a complete healthy lifestyle will provide you with more energy, more mental alertness, more living out of your years, and more years out of your living.

These 3 foods have been selected for this book from the thousands of very nourishing foods offered in Nature for very specific reasons. They are all:
1) inexpensive, costing pennies per day
2) widely available, in the city or country, warm or cold climate
3) extraordinary healing agents, with both scientific documentation and centuries of folk medicine to support their use
4) very versatile, and can help a wide assortment of seemingly unrelated problems
5) very safe, especially when compared to the risk: benefit ratio of prescription drugs

6) blessed with an incredibly long shelf life, when properly stored

❀PERSONAL PROFILE: MY EXPERIENCES

I was born on a farm in Illinois. My grandfather was a corn and cattle farmer all of his life. He brushed his teeth with baking soda and never had a cavity nor lost a tooth. My mother has always had an uncommon appreciation for "keeping it simple" and appreciating Nature. Combine these traits with my natural curiosity that surfaced early in life as I took apart 5 different watches that were given to me, tried making my own battery recharger before there was such a thing, and even dissected worms in my spare time. I needed to know "what makes things tick". After studying both science and folk medicine extensively, I can tell you that a "mysterious force", sometimes called Nature makes everything "tick". When we cooperate with that Force and provide it with the proper raw materials, things "tick" well, even though we don't understand why.

Over the 18 years of my career as a professional clinical nutritionist, I have found more and more "simple solutions for complex modern health problems". Knowing what makes people "tick" has helped in the biochemistry of my profession and in better understanding people's behavior. Oftentimes, these simple solutions were not widely known because there was no international pharmaceutical company to champion the marketing campaign.

About 10 years ago, I began to research and use folk medicine for myself and my wife, Noreen. We both have had some noteworthy successes. My frequent urination was cured through the use of apple cider vinegar, a remedy found later in the chapter on vinegar. My occasional upset stomach was cured by taking a spoonful of raw honey at night on an empty stomach. By adding considerable garlic to our diet, from a special "no odor" recipe, we have dramatically boosted our energy levels and reduced our bouts with colds and flu. We are usually healthy, even when working around sick patients and playing around lots of sick children. We have used honey as a topically applied antibiotic to prevent infections on cuts. We use vinegar to cleanse the pesticides off of fresh produce. We use many of the remedies and recipes found in this book; and we are real believers in the healing, energizing, and cleansing power of these superfoods.

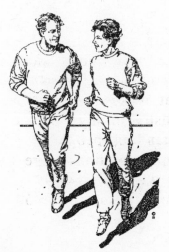

So sit back with a cup of your favorite beverage, relax, and enjoy some stories, some facts, some remedies, and some recipes on how Nature and science have cooperated to provide you with 3 superfoods that will supercharge your life in more ways than you can imagine.

Chapter 2

📖

HONEY FACTS & REMEDIES

Sweet healer from Nature's bosom

"The Doctor of the future will give no medicine, but will involve the patient in the proper use of food, fresh air, and exercise." Thomas Edison, celebrated inventor

A TOUCH OF HONEY

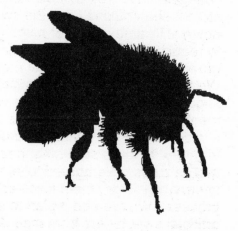

A touch of honey, a
touch of love;
A touch from
Someone's hand above.

A touch of sweetness,
in bread and wine,
A touch of honey
makes the common
sublime.

A touch of honey in muffin and scone;
Make the honey touch your own!

Sweetness to pancakes, biscuits and toast,
Sweetness to drinks, even halibut roast.

A touch of honey, gift of the bee,
Gathered from flowers for you and me.
by Doris Mech

❀ PERSONAL PROFILE. MT was a busy working mom with 3 kids. At ages 3, 6 and 12, the kids each had unique taste buds. One thing was certain, though: they all had a sweet tooth, just like their mother. MT noticed the amount of diet soft drinks that she was buying was becoming a serious portion of her grocery bill. She also had read some disturbing news that artificial sweeteners may not be as safe as we all once thought. Her oldest child was starting the dieting phase of teen years. Her next child was becoming a white sugar addict and had a miserable report card from the dentist to support his problem. The youngest child would throw temper tantrums in the grocery store if she couldn't have the sweets that she wanted right now. MT came to me for help. I explained to her the need to regulate blood sugar levels in order to have proper growth and optimal levels of mental and physical energy. We talked about the irreversible deterioration started when sugar rots adult teeth. For her diet soda addiction, I mentioned how aspartame has been reportedly linked with a wide variety of nervous disorders, including loss of memory, labored breathing, headaches, and even grand mal seizures. We agreed to let the kids in on this important information to get them involved in the decision making process. We created a plan to slowly remove sugar and artificial sweeteners from their diet and replace it with much less honey. The kids became very attached to the taste of honey, and while it is more expensive than white sugar, mom noticed that the grocery bills went down considerably when the family started making their own beverages (recipes found in the next chapter) with honey rather than consuming all that diet pop. Once the family replaced unhealthy sweeteners with the healthiest sweetener of all, honey, the kids health improved, grades went up, disagreements went down, and dentist bills were non-existent. MT was very happy with the improvements that honey had made in her home.

The bee is a true marvel of nature. Based upon the principles that we use to build airplanes, or aeronautical engineering, bees should not be able to fly. Along with silkworms, bees are the only domesticated insects on earth, creating vast reserves of bee's wax, honey, bee pollen, and royal jelly. Without bees we would lose the 2.2 billion pounds of annual honey production around the world. Without the cross pollination that bees provide in their pollen and nectar gathering, there would be at least 90 species of fruits, vegetables, and grains that would die out. Without bees, history would not have included wax candles to light up the night, wax molds to make gold ornaments, references to "love as sweet as honey", and the many major decisions inspired by mead wine.

Honey was so valuable to our ancestors that Romans used it in place of gold to pay their taxes. Notice that "money" and "honey" differ only by one letter. Greek athletes would eat honey before entering the arena of competition. In the Old Testament, Jacob sent an offering of honey to Joseph, the ruler of Egypt to generate good feelings. In the great Egyptian civilization which created the Pyramids, honey was given to children to ward off evil spirits and buried in tombs as a food for the hereafter. Jars of honey have been found in Egyptian tombs 3300 years after they were buried--and the honey was still edible!! Most "junk food" has a long shelf life because bacteria cannot survive off this stuff, while honey has an even longer shelf life because of antibiotic agents to halt bacterial growth, which were created by the bees.

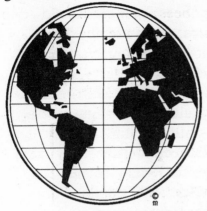

Americans eat an average of 285 million pounds of honey each year, which is only possible because the average bee hive produces 3 times more honey than the bees need to survive. To pollinate California's approximately 360,000 bearing acres of almonds, it is estimated that 250,000 colonies of honey bees must be borrowed from other states to add to the 500,000 colonies already in the state. It takes 556 worker bees flying 35,584 miles (1.3 times around the world) to produce one pound of honey! Which means that 1.2 trillion bees fly a total of 80 trillion miles to produce the world's annual honey supply. Compare that distance flown to the 90 million miles from the earth to the sun. The average life of a worker bee is 6 weeks, at which time the bee's wings are worn to shreds and the bee dies of exhaustion.

Some nutritionists would argue that honey is nothing more than another simple carbohydrate, like white sugar. Actually, honey is a complex collection of enzymes, plant pigments, organic acids, esters, antibiotic agents, trace minerals like chromium, and other unidentified nutrition factors. Since honey is a partially digested product from the bees gut, the digestive enzymes probably play an important role in the nutritional value of honey. Therefore, always use "raw" or "unpasteurized" honey, since cooking the honey denatures its valuable enzymes. If you are going to cook with honey, you can use the cheaper commercial pasteurized products.

Realize that honey is a combination of nectar, which is the sweet syrup produced by flowers to attract bees for their cross-pollination talents, plus the pollen, which is the plant equivalent of human sperm; all of which has been digested in the bees gut. Thus, honey is a teeming collection of very metabolically active nutrient factors.

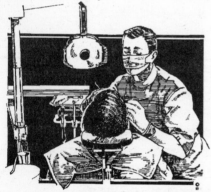

While white sugar clearly is a major factor generating cavities in Western society, raw honey does not fuel cavity-making bacteria with the same fervor. In animal studies, honey did not create erosion of tooth enamel, as would be expected based upon its sticky sugar content.[1] This is probably because honey contains a collection of antibiotic agents, which would stop the bacteria in the mouth from using sugar to erode the tooth enamel.

While refined white sugar, or sucrose, can dramatically raise blood sugar levels, which can be lethal to diabetics and is unhealthy for everyone; honey does not raise blood glucose as high, giving it a more favorable "glycemic" index and making

honey the preferred sweetener in the kitchen
PERIOD.

About 75% of the weight of honey is the
simple sugars of dextrose (glucose) and fructose
(levulose). Most other essential nutrients are also
present in small quantities.

One pound (453 grams) of honey contains:
**1333 calories (compared to one pound of white
sugar containing 1748 calories)**
1.4 grams of protein
23 mg (milligrams) of calcium
73 mg of phosphorus
4.1 mg of iron
1.0 mg of niacin
16 mg of vitamin C

Bees are not only hard working nectar
"farmers", but they are also connoisseurs of fine
flower nectar, and quite vulnerable to toxins such
as pesticide spray. Which means that honey is
usually gathered from the sweetest of nearby
flowers and is free of contamination from
dangerous sprays.

There are as many different types of honey as
there are combinations of bee strains and plants
with nectar. Of the 20,000 different species of bees
(Apoidea), most are solitary and thus do not gather
extra honey for human harvesting. Yet, there are
over 200 different types of honey harvested in the
United States alone, with clover honey accounting
for 70% of sales.

Certain regions of America have developed their own regional favorites, such as orange blossom honey from California, buckwheat honey from New York, tupelo honey from Florida, and fireweed honey from Washington. The Puget Sound area of northwest Washington state has some unique honeys, including maple blossom, raspberry, wild blackberry, wild huckleberry, and snowberry. As you become more enthused about honey, you may start looking for small local apiaries (bee hives) and develop your own connoiseur tastes with the many variations of honey!!

> **"I eat my peas with honey**
> **I've done it all my life;**
> **It makes the peas taste funny,**
> **But keeps them on my knife!"**

BEE PRODUCTS

•Honey is the sweet liquid produced by bees from the nectar of flowers. The color and flavor of the honey will be determined by the source of the nectar. Most of the honey produced in the United States is from clover or alfalfa, which produces light-colored and delicately flavored honeys. Much of the commercial honey is a blend of several honeys.

Honey is harvested in the form of comb honey, which may be cut in squares and sold. More often, the honey is strained out of the comb, pasteurized (cooked), and then bottled as a clear liquid. The whitish, opaque, creamed honey is actually honey that has been crystallized. Because honey has the ability to absorb moisture, it is often used in the baking industry to keep baked goods moist and fresh. Its high sugar content and its acidity make it an excellent food preservative.

•Propolis. Bees gather the sap from certain trees for its antibacterial properties. This "propolis", from the Greek word meaning "defenses before the town", contains a natural antibiotic, called galangin, and is used to line the hive to prevent the buildup of bacteria and viruses. Propolis, sold in health food stores, is often taken as an immune stimulant, used for thymus enhancement, and added to cosmetics. People who do not like to take antibiotics use propolis to treat low grade infections.

•Bee Pollen. As worker bees gather nectar, their hind legs collect the pollen from the plant's flower. Hive keepers are able to harvest this pollen by placing a wire mesh entrance at the hive. As the bees struggle to get through this narrow entry, the pollen falls into a collecting basket below. Bee pollen, which is up to 35% protein, is used in energy drinks and bars and for a wide assortment of ailments, including allergy relief.

•Royal bee jelly. There is a fascinating caste system in bee hives. While worker bees live only about 6 weeks, the queen bee lasts up to 9 years. Worker bees are female bees that are not allowed to hatch eggs. Worker bees gather a unique collection of pollen, nectar, and plant resins to create royal bee jelly, which is fed only to the queen bee for fertility and long life. This nutrient-rich substance contains all of the essential amino acids, special fatty acids, all the B vitamins with special emphasis on pantothenic acid; as well as the minerals iron, potassium, calcium, silicon, and sulfur. Royal jelly helps to treat fatigue, insomnia, ulcers, digestive disorders, and cardiovascular ailments.

•Mead. Making alcoholic drinks basically involves fermenting some carbohydrate food; such as grapes for wine, rice for saki, and so on. Honey is the primary carbohydrate food that is used to make the legendary mead wine, which influenced much of our ancient history, until grape growers found an easier way to gather sugary foods.

BEES: THE ULTIMATE WORKERS

Beekeeping, or apiculture, is the cultivation of colonies of honeybees. Commercial beekeeping includes the production of honey and beeswax, the breeding of bees for sale, and the rental of bees for pollinating crops. Beekeeping in most of the world means cultivating the western honeybee, Apis mellifera. The infamous killer bee, a relative of the African honeybee, is too aggressive for commercial beekeeping.   Modern beekeeping is based on the ancient Greek technique of creating a bee space. In those days, the hive consisted of a basket containing a series of parallel wooden bars separated by a distance equal to that between honeycombs when they are naturally built by bees. That distance is 6.350 millimeters, or about one quarter of an inch. Any variation from this distance results in the space being filled with comb or propolis. A honeycomb is a mass of hexagonal cells in the nest that contain eggs, young bees, and honey.

Lorenzo Lorraine Langstroth in 1851 brought beekeeping to the United States. The typical beehive today comprises a bottom board and several boxes containing movable frames and a cover. Each frame is furnished with a beeswax foundation imprinted with the hexagonal shapes of cell bottoms. The bees are guided by the imprinted cells in building their honeycombs.

The world's annual production of more than 2.2 billion pounds of honey could be replaced with other sugar products, but the services of honeybees as pollinators of some 90 crops would be lost. Due to today's more efficient single-crop agribusiness, there has been little or no grassland where bees can find nesting sites or weeds that supply nectar and pollen. The use of pesticides to control harmful insects has also reduced the population of beneficial insects such as bees.

Today, fruit and seed growers contract with beekeepers to move honeybee colonies onto the farms. This "bee herding" ensures income to the beekeeper during years when honey production drops off. With the moving of the hives comes the risk of spreading American foulbrood, a disease that can wipe out a hive. Some beekeepers routinely feed antibiotics to their bees to avoid losses from infections. In the first season there will probably not be a honey harvest because an average hive requires 90 lb (40 kg) of honey to survive the winter.

Bees belong to the same order as wasps. Like wasps, bees have mouth parts adapted for both chewing and sucking, but the bee's tongue is longer than the wasp's and better suited for gathering nectar from a greater variety of flowers. Bees have feathery body hairs, also known as plumose. Females have brushes on their legs, and they use these brushes to remove pollen that sticks to the body hairs. The pollen is then stored under the abdomen or on the hind legs.

Bees are subdivided into several families on the basis of how their wings are veined, and other criteria. Most of the 20,000 species are solitary bees. There are many unique species of bees, some of which live in the ground and a few even eat wood. One of the more fascinating bees, the giant Indian bee (Apis dorsata) builds a single comb as large as 5 feet by 3 feet (1.5 x 1 meter) attached to rocks, trees, or buildings. There are people in India who specialize in harvesting this honey by smoking out the bees from these hives that are built on high cliffs. Since the honey is so difficult to gather, these people do not consume anywhere near the 132 pounds per year of sugar that their American counterparts do.

Bee are extremely hard working creatures with a very rigid social order. The entire efforts of the worker (infertile females) and drone (males) bees are all geared toward serving the needs of the queen bee, who is the pivotal point for the survival of the hive. Drones are extremely disposable in the bee hive, with the exception of fertilizing eggs for the queen bee at certain times of the year. Drones develop from unfertilized eggs that the queen produces by withholding sperm from the eggs laid in large drone cells. Drones lack stingers and the structures needed for pollen collection. In the autumn they are ejected by the colony to starve, unless the colony is queenless. New drones are produced in the spring for mating.

Female larvae also may be evicted from the hive to control the population. When the female workers lay eggs, the queen may chase the workers away and eat the eggs; but if the queen dies or is removed, one of the larger workers will take her place within four hours or less. The difference in size of workers is dependent upon the amount of food they have available to eat when they are larvae.

Both queens and workers are produced from fertilized eggs. Queen larvae are reared in special peanut-shaped cells and fed more of the pharyngeal gland secretions of the nurse bees, also called bee milk or royal bee jelly. Although workers are similar in appearance and behavior to other female bees, they lack the structures for mating. When no queen is present to inhibit the development of their ovaries, however, workers eventually begin to lay eggs that develop into drones.

When a new queen is needed for the hive, the first queen to emerge stings the other queens before they have a chance to mature. Within a few days, the virgin queen will fly to where drones assemble, and mate with 6 to 12 drones. The sperm from these drones is stored in a sac and used during her egg-laying life of from two to nine years.

When queens fly to mate, a pheromone (special scent) attracts the drones. The same gland produces another pheromone, called queen substance, which workers lick from the queen's body and pass along as they exchange food with one another. The eaten pheromone keeps the other female workers infertile. When the queen's secretion is inadequate, the colony produces queen cells to take over.

Colonies kept in hives yield an average of 50 pounds (23 kg) of honey for the beekeeper. Unlike other bees, honeybees do not hibernate during cold weather. They survive the rigors of northern winters by feeding on stored supplies and sharing their body heat, clustering together in dense packs.

Bees are world class navigators. Honeybees communicate direction and distance from the hive to nectar sources through a sophisticated dance "language". In 1973, Karl von Frisch received a Nobel Prize for deciphering this bee language, which consists of a circle dance and a tail-wagging dance; which accurately tells other bees the angle from the sun and distance to the nectar. Bees use the sun as a compass, orienting the dance angle to the plane of sunlight. Even when the sun is obscured by clouds, bees can detect its position from the light in brighter patches of the sky.

Bees also can see ultraviolet designs in flowers like an airplane circling Dallas airport observes the landing lights on the runway. Honeybees also have a built-in clock that appears to be synchronized with the secretion of nectar from flowers. Thus, honeybees making the rounds of flowers in search of nectar always seem to be in the right place at the right time.

EXAMPLES OF "HONEY" REFERENCES IN THE BIBLE:

Genesis 43:11	a little balm, and a little honey
Exodus 3:8	flowing with milk and honey;
16:31	like wafers made with honey.
Leviticus 2:11	burn no leaven, nor any honey
Numbers 13:27	floweth with milk and honey;
Deut 6:3	floweth with milk and honey.
8:8	a land of oil olive and honey;
Joshua 5:6	floweth with milk and honey.
Judges 14:8	bees and honey
9	honey out of the carcass
18	What is sweeter than honey?
1 Samuel 14:25	honey upon the ground.
26	the honey dropped
29	I tasted a little of this honey.
43	taste a little honey
2 Samuel 17:29	And honey, and butter
2 Kings 18:32	a land of oil olive and of honey
2 Chron 31:5	wine, and oil, and honey, and
Job 20:17	floods, the brooks of honey
Psalm 19:10	gold: sweeter also than honey
81:16	and with honey out of the rock
119:103	sweeter than honey to my mouth
Proverbs 24:13	eat the honey, because it is good
25:16	found honey
27	not good to eat much honey
Solomon 4:11	honey and milk

5:1	eaten my honeycomb
Isaac 7:15	Butter and honey shall he eat
22	honey shall every one eat
Jeremiah 11:5	flowing with milk and honey
41:8	and of honey.
Ezekiel 3:3	as honey for sweetness.
16:13	didst eat fine flour, and honey
Matthew 3:4	locusts and wild honey.
Rev 10:9	sweet as honey.

REMEDIES
"Natural forces within us are the true healers."
Hippocrates, father of modern medicine, 400 B.C.

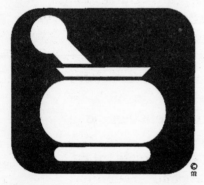

STOMACH PROBLEMS. For acid indigestion, take 1-3 teaspoons of honey. For chronic problems, take 1 tablespoon of honey at bedtime on an empty stomach. Scientists now find that a major cause of dyspepsia (upset stomach) is the bacteria strain, Helicobacter pylori. A 5% solution of honey completely inhibited the growth of all 7 strains of Helicobacter in petri dishes.[2] Honey has been a longstanding champion recommended by savvy doctors even in the noted medical journal, Lancet, for the treatment of ulcers.[3]

WOUND HEALER. Because honey is rich in sugar, enzymes, vitamins, minerals, and other nutrient factors, it has become an unsurpassed healer when applied topically to wounds. Not only does honey protect the wound from infections while providing nutrients for the wound to begin the repair process, but honey also seems to be superior to more expensive hospital wound dressings. In a study published in the British Journal of Plastic Surgery, researchers randomly assigned 46 burn patients to either get honey in the wound dressing or a hospital product called OpSite. Honey provided for faster wound healing.[4] Another group of Australian researchers found that honey topically applied accelerated wound recovery in women who had Caesarean deliveries.[5] In dealing with a nasty type of gangrene (Fournier's), physicians found that honey applied to the affected area eliminated the need for surgery and anesthesia. There were no deaths in the honey group versus 3 (out of 21 patients) deaths in the group that received routine antibiotics and wound dressing.[6] Honey is no longer just folk medicine, it is the medicine of choice in many health situations.

INFANT SOOTHER. Use honey in infant formulas to provide a wholesome sweetener, supplementary minerals, an antiseptic, and a mild laxative. It also has a definite beneficial influence upon calcium retention.

WEIGHT LOSS. Honey used as a sweetener does not result in heavy production of body fat as does refined sugar. It is palatable and digestible as well as nutritious.

ATHLETIC PERFORMANCE. Many nutrition experts consider honey excellent nourishment, a "power supply" for the heart muscle. To make your own "Gatorade" type beverage, add 3 tablespoons of honey (or to taste), plus 1 teaspoon of Lite Salt (which is half potassium), plus 1 tablespoon of apple cider vinegar to one quart of purified water. Drink often when sweating.

ANTISEPTIC & ANTIBIOTIC. Besides being a superb energy food, honey is one of nature's most powerful germ killers. Germs simply cannot survive in honey. Primitive man not only used honey as food, but also as medicine to heal his wounds.

LAXATIVE. Honey is a natural laxative, and one of the fastest working stimulants known.

FACIAL TREATMENT

1/3 c. finely ground oatmeal
3 t. honey, or enough to make a smooth paste
1 t. rose water or orange flower water
Blend oatmeal with honey until well mixed. If too thick and unmanageable, add a little rose water or orange flower water. Spread over clean face with the exception of your eyes and leave on for 1/2 hour. Relax while it is on. Remove with soft washcloth and warm water. Following this, a good astringent should be applied to tone the skin.

FACE LOTION

1 T. sweet almond oil
2 T. honey
Blend together. This lotion should be used after the skin has been thoroughly cleansed. It should be permitted to remain on the skin about 1/2 hour. Remove it with a soft cloth and tepid water. Following this, apply milk astringent to close the pores and tone the skin.

FACIAL SOFTENING
1/4 t. apple cider vinegar
1 T. honey
Beat well and spread liberally over the face. Leave on for 15 minutes and rinse off in warm water. Pat dry.

FACIAL BALM FROM CLEOPATRA
1 t. honey
1 egg white
1 t. milk
Beat well and apply to clean face and neck. Leave on 1/2 hour. When it feels dry and brittle, wash it off with lukewarm water. Splash on cold water. You will feel your face and neck tingle. Cleopatra used this formula on her entire body to keep her skin soft and young looking.

EYE MAGIC FORMULA
1 T. honey
1 egg white
Mix well and with the fingertips pat the mixture into the tissue around the eyes.
Do not pull on the skin. Always
use a gentle patting motion when
touching this area. Allow time for
the honey & egg white mixture to
dry. Then wash off gently with
warm water. Does wonders for
tightening up the skin around the
eye area.

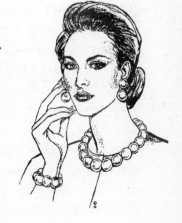

FACIAL SCRUB
1/2 c. almond meal
Honey
Mix to form a thick paste. Scrub

face with paste, paying close attention to oily areas where black heads or blemishes occur and being careful to avoid the area of your eyes. Leave on for a few minutes. Remove with tepid water and a soft cloth. Your skin will be soft and refreshed.

HAND SCRUB

3 T. finely ground corn meaL
1 t. cornstarch
2 T. honey

Blend corn meal and cornstarch and add honey. Place in a small jar. Use as you would any hand soap. It softens, cleans and smoothes the hands. Always rinse hands with cold water.

ELBOW RUB SOFTENER

1 t. lemon juice
1 t. cold pressed safflower oil
1 t. honey

Beat well until thoroughly blended. Rub mixture onto elbows and massage for a few minutes. A stubborn case of muddy looking, dry elbow skin can be helped considerably by frequent applications. If used often, you will notice a lightening of the skin tone in this area, plus a new resiliency to the skin and a softening of the previously hard surface.

BURN CURE FROM GRANDMA

1 egg yolk
Honey
1 T. olive oil

Mix these ingredients thoroughly together. Spread on a surgical gauze and place on the burn. When the dressing dries, repeat the treatment until the healing is complete. The pain should subside and disappear completely.

OLD COUNTRY OINTMENT

1 part flour
1 part honey
Mix together. Apply on wounds or skin troubles.
Variation: Add propolis, the gummy substance
exuded by trees such as is found on the scales
protecting the leaf buds of horse chestnuts in
spring.

DIARRHEA CURE

1 t. honey
8 oz. barley water
Mix honey in barley water and drink. This will stop
summer diarrhea.

BEDWETTING TREATMENT

For at least 3 hours before bedtime, make sure that
the child does not get any liquids. At bedtime, give
he or she a tablespoon of honey, followed by
brushing the teeth.

TRANQUILIZER

1 c. chamomile tea
Fresh or dry mint leaves
1 t. honey
Steep 3 minutes. Drink before going to bed. You'll
sleep well.

COUGH SYRUP

1 t. honey
1 t. lemon juice
Mix equal proportions of honey and lemon juice and
use as needed for simple cough.

COUGH SYRUP

1/4 c. spicy honey
1 T. pure glycerine
1 T. fresh lime or lemon juice

Purchase glycerine at your drugstore. Blend well. Keep in a covered jar and take 1 teaspoon every 2 hours or as needed.

SORE THROAT REMEDY

2 t. buckwheat honey
2 t. glycerine
2 t. lemon juice
1/2 t. powdered ginger

Combine and heat in a jar over hot water. When well blended, remove from heat and shake jar vigorously. Sip a teaspoonful slowly at night before going to bed. It will soothe your throat. Use warm or at room temperature.

MAGIC TONIC

2 t. honey
1 glass water
2 t. apple cider vinegar

Mix together and drink once a day for enhanced energy, better disease resistance, and clearer mind.

HONEY EGG TONIC

3 T. mild honey
1 egg yolk
2 T. butter
Dash of salt

Beat until smooth and creamy. Store in a jar, tightly covered, in refrigerator. Spread 1 tablespoonful of mixture on hot toast or biscuit. Eat about 15 minutes before breakfast and supper. Repeat several weeks or until you feel better.

SPRING TONIC

1 c. honey
sulphur powder

Purchase sulphur powder at your drugstore. Mix powder with honey to make a thick paste. Take 1 teaspoon before breakfast for 21 days at the beginning of spring. Good cleanser and energizer for all.

---

[1]. Grobbler, SR, et al., Archives of Oral Biology, vol.39, no.2, p.147, Feb.1994

[2]. al Somal, N, et al., JR Society of Medicine, vol.87, no.1, p.9, Jan.1994

[3]. Postmes, T, et al, Lancet, vol.341, p.756, Mar.20, 1993; see also Greenwood, D, Lancet, vol.341, p.90, Jan.9, 1993

[4]. Subrahmanyam, M, British Journal of Plastic Surgery, vol.46, no.4, p.322, June 1993

[5]. Phuapradit, W. et al., Australia & New Zealand Journal of Obstetrics and Gynaecology, vol.32, no.4, p.381, Nov.1992

[6]. Efem, SE, Surgery, vol.113, no.2, p.200, Feb.1993

Chapter 3

📖

HONEY RECIPES

cooking with Nature's sweetest ingredient

Mine be a cot beside the hill;
A beehive's hum shall soothe my ear;
A willowy brook that turns a mill,
With many a fall shall linger near.
-Samuel Rogers 1763-1855

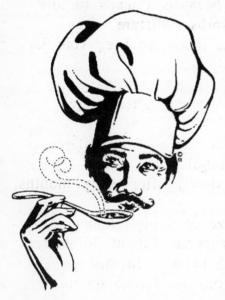

❀ PERSONAL PROFILE. KL was a busy housewife with grown kids to be proud of. She stayed involved in various groups and travelled with her husband extensively. But she had allergies to all kinds of things. From pollen and ragweed, to milk and wheat. Some doctors told her there were more food that she was allergic to than she could eat. She did not like taking the medication which was prescribed for her allergies, since it made her drousy. KL came to me for help. We worked on a sensible program to remove most of the dairy from her diet, including cheeses and milk. It is almost impossible to eat in a restaurant without getting some milk products in your diet. I suggested that she have her many mercury fillings replaced with non-metal composites. Mercury poisoning is widespread, especially in people with mercury amalgams.

Mercury can create immune disorders which include hypersensitivity to allergens. I put KL on a regular supplement program of vitamin C, selenium, fish oil, and bee pollen. Bee pollen can be extremely helpful in subduing the symptoms of allergies. Within 3 weeks, her sneezing and red eyes had gone away and within 12 weeks, KL reported no more allergic symptoms. She was free to enjoy her busy and exciting life.

GENERAL GUIDELINES FOR COOKING WITH HONEY

When substituting honey for sugar in your own recipes, follow these general guidelines.

Cover honey tightly because it tends to lose aroma and flavor and absorbs moisture when exposed to air. Insects like it too, so keep your jar lid clean or you may attract ants.

Foods sweetened with honey will have a better flavor if kept until the day after baking before it is served.

Freezing does not injure the color of flavor of honey, but may hasten granulation.

Honey may darken slowly after many months, but it will still be usable.

Honey will caramelize at a high temperature, so use a lower oven temperature (about 30 degrees F. lower) when baking with honey. In this way, a cake or bread cannot become too brown on top before it is done on the inside.

Honey's acidity is a natural asset. However, to neutralize honey's natural acidity, add 1/12 teaspoon of baking soda to the ingredients per cup of honey. When sour milk is used with honey in a recipe, you may omit the extra soda.

If you're baking desserts for to be stored or shipped, honey will help your baked goods stay oven fresh because of its marvelous "keeping" qualities.

Keep honey in a warm, dry place where you would keep salt. Room temperature, 70 to 80 degrees F. is best.

Lower baking temperature 25 to 30 degrees F. to prevent overbrowning.

Store honey at room temperature, not in the refrigerator. Keep container closed tightly and in a dry place.

Substitute 3/4 cup honey for 1 cup sugar. Reduce total amount of other liquids by 1/4 cup per cup of honey.

To bring crystallized honey back to its natural liquid state, place container of honey in a pan of warm water until crystals disappear.

When using honey in cooking, moisten the measuring spoon or cup first with water or oil, then measure the honey. This will eliminate sticking.

Drinks

SWEET COFFEE
1/3 C. milk
1 rounded tsp. honey
2/3 C. strong coffee

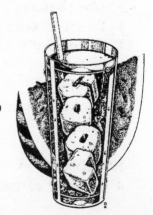

Fill your blender with hot tap water. Microwave milk and honey in a coffee mug for 30 seconds on high. Fill the mug up with hot coffee. Empty water out of the blender and process coffee and milk for about 30 seconds until foamy. Pour into mug and top with a dash of cocoa or cinnamon, if desired.

PEPPERMINT FIZZ
1/4 C. chopped fresh peppermint leaves
1 tsp. honey
2/3 C. boiling water
Juice of 1 orange
Juice of 1 lemon
1 C. sparkling mineral water or soda water
6 ice cubes
1 lg. sprig mint, to decorate
   Put the chopped mint in a quart-sized pre-warmed jar. Pour on the boiling water and stir in the honey. Cover and allow to cool, then add the freshly squeezed fruit juices. Chill in the refrigerator for 2 or 3 hours, then strain and add the sparkling water. Pour in glasses with ice cubes. Decorate each glass with a little sprig of fresh mint and serve immediately.

BANANA HEALTH SHAKE
1 ripe banana
1 T. dried skim milk
1 T. brewer's yeast
1 T. honey
1 c. milk
   Mix thoroughly in a blender until smooth and creamy.

HONEY COCOA
4 t. cocoa or carob

1/3 c. hot water
4 to 5 t. honey
Few grains of salt
1 1/3 c. milk

Mix the cocoa, honey, salt, and water in a pan. Cook, stirring constantly, until the mixture boils. Continue to cook for about 2 minutes. Place over hot water and stir in the milk. Heat thoroughly. Serves 2.

READY LEMONADE
1 c. lemon juice
1/2 c. honey

Mix well and keep in refrigerator in tightly covered jar. To each 1/4 cup of the sweetened lemon juice, add 1 cup ice water for lemonade anytime.

HONEY FRUIT PUNCH
1 qt. boiling water
1 1/4 t. black tea
5 whole cloves
1 c. orange juice
1 qt. lime juice
1/2 c. lemon juice
1/2 c. liquid honey
1 c. cold water

Pour boiling water over tea and cloves. Let steep 5 minutes. Combine tea with the other ingredients; pour over ice to chill. Garnish with orange slices or mint leaves. Makes 24 servings.

HONEY ICE CUBES
Blend:
1/2 c. honey
2 c. very hot water
2 T. lemon juice
　　Freeze. Good for ice tea and punch.

Vegetables

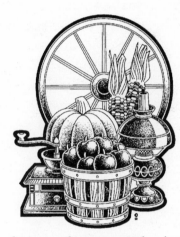

CITRUS HONEY CARROTS
1 bunch carrots
1 pinch of salt
1/4 c. melted butter
1/4 c. honey
1 1/2 t. grated orange peel
1 1/2 t. grated lemon peel
　　Wash and scrape carrots. Steam carrots until crispy tender, about 15 to 20 minutes; drain. Blend melted butter, honey and citrus peels. Pour over cooked carrots and place over low heat until carrots are thoroughly glazed. Makes 4 servings.

SWEET POTATO DELIGHT
2 (16 oz.) cans sweet potatoes (in heavy syrup), drained
2 large apples, peeled, cored and cut into 1/4 inch slices
1/4 c. chopped walnuts
1/2 c. dark seedless raisins
1/2 c. honey

1 t. grated orange peel
1/2 t. salt
1/8 t. mace
1/8 t. ground ginger
1/4 c. butter

Cut sweet potatoes into 1/2 inch slices. Layer
in a lightly greased 1 1/2 quart casserole with
apple slices, raisins and walnuts. Combine honey,
butter, orange peel, salt, cinnamon, and ginger in a
saucepan. Heat until margarine is melted and
mixture is well blended. Pour over layered sweet
potatoes and fruits. Bake, uncovered, at 350
degrees for about 1 hour, basting occasionally.
Serves 8..

HONEY ACORN SQUASH
1 acorn squash
2 t. honey
1/4 t. salt
1/8 t. pepper
1/8 t. mace
1 t. butter

Cut squash in half lengthwise and remove
seeds. Place in baking pan with 1/2 inch water
covering bottom of pan. Spread honey over inside
squash. Add seasonings and butter. Cover; bake in
moderate oven, 350 degrees for about 1 hour.
Uncover; brown top delicately. Serves 2.

SCALLOPED TOMATOES
1 can tomatoes, stewed
2 T. butter
2 T. honey

1 c. whole wheat cracker crumbs
1/2 t. salt
Pepper to taste
Drain liquid from tomatoes. Cover bottom of buttered baking dish with a layer of tomatoes. Sprinkle with salt, pepper, dots of butter, and honey. Cover with a layer of cracker crumbs. Repeat with another layer of tomatoes, crumbs and seasoning. Bake at 400 degrees for 20 minutes.

Salads with honey

CABBAGE SESAME SALAD
1 C. finely sliced red cabbage
1 C. finely sliced white cabbage
1 or 2 sliced green onions
1 T. fresh parsley, finely chopped
2 T. sesame seeds
A few spinach leaves
1/4 C. oil canola oi!
2 T. honey
1/4 C. vinegar
Marinate the red and white cabbage with the onions and parsley in the oil-honey-vinegar mixture for at least 10 minutes in the refrigerator. Serve with a slotted spoon, placing individual portions on a bed of spinach leaves. Sprinkle with sesame seeds.

FRESH SPINACH SALAD
2 bunches of fresh spinach
1/2 lb. fresh mung bean sprouts
6 slices turkey bacon, fried and crumbled

3 hard-boiled eggs, chopped

Toss all the ingredients together in a large salad bowl. Serve immediately with the honey dressing. Serves 8.

Honey dressing:
1/2 C. canola oil
1/3 C. honey
1/4 C. catsup
1/3 C. apple cider vinegar
1 T. Worcestershire sauce
1 med. sweet white onion, chopped

Mix the oil, honey, catsup, vinegar and Worcestershire sauce together in blender until smooth. Stir in the onion. Refrigerate.

GARBANZO SALAD
15 oz. can garbanzo beans, drained
14 1/2 oz. can stewed tomato pieces, drained
1/4 C. chopped green pepper
1/4 C. red onion, sliced
2 T. currants
pepper
1 T. parsley
3 T. tomato sauce
1 T. honey

Combine the garbanzo beans, tomatoes, green pepper, onion, currants, pepper and parsley. Stir the tomato sauce together with the honey in a cup. Mix all the ingredients.

MARINATED VEGETABLES
1 lg. carrot, cut in strips
1 green onion, sliced

1 C. broccoli flowerets
1/2 cucumber, sliced
1/2 C. red cabbage, sliced
1/2 C. tomato, sliced
 Marinate in the following mixture and place in the refrigerator.
Marinade:
1/4 C. oil
2 T. honey
1/4 C. vinegar
 Blend together.

CARROT RAISIN SALAD
3 c. grated raw carrots
1 c. seedless raisins
1 T. honey
6 T. plain yogurt
1/4 c. milk
1 T. fresh lemon juice
1/4 t. salt
1/4 t. nutmeg
 Toss carrots with raisins. Blend remaining ingredients and stir into carrot mixture. Chill.
Serves 6.

GOLDEN SALAD
1 pkg. lemon gelatin
1 c. boiling water
3/4 c. pineapple juice
2 T. lemon juice
1 T. honey
1/4 t. salt
3/4 c. grated raw carrots

1/2 c. crushed, canned pineapple, well drained
Dissolve gelatin in boiling water to which salt had been added. Add pineapple juice, lemon juice and honey. Mix well and add raw carrots and pineapple. Pour into mold which has been rinsed in cold water. When thoroughly set, unmold, arrange on lettuce leaf, and garnish. Serves 8.

BANANA NUT AMBROSIA
2 bananas, cut crosswise
2 T. honey
1 T. pineapple juice
1/4 c. chopped nuts
1/4 c. shredded coconut
1/4 c. yogurt
Arrange sliced bananas on greens. Mix yogurt, honey and juice and spoon over fruit. Sprinkle nuts and coconut on top.

SNAPPY HONEY SALAD DRESSING
1/2 c. honey
1/2 t. salt
1/3 c. chili sauce
1 T. grated onion
1 T. Worcestershire sauce
1/2 c. canola oil
1/3 c. vinegar
Combine honey, salt, chili sauce, vinegar, onion, and Worcestershire sauce. Slowly add the salad oil, beating until well blended.

FRUIT DRESSING
1/2 c. yogurt

1 T. honey
1 t. grated lemon peel
2 T. non-fat cream cheese
1 T. lemon juice
        Combine honey, lemon juice, peel, and cheese. Mix with yogurt.

HONEY CHEESE DRESSING
1/2 c. cottage cheese
2 T. honey
1 t. grated lemon rind
1 1/4 T. lemon juice
1/2 t. salt
1/3 c canola oil
        Force cottage cheese through a sieve. Add honey, lemon rind, juice, and salt. Beat briskly with an egg beater. Add oil, a teaspoon at a time, until well blended.

COLE SLAW DRESSING
1 c. non-fat sour cream
1/2 c. honey
Dash of salt
Juice of 1 lemon (or lime)
        Beat all together until well blended. Chill.

UNCOOKED APPLESAUCE
3 lg. apples
1 qt. cold water
1 T. lemon juice
1/4 tsp. cinnamon or nutmeg
1/4 C. honey

Wash the apples. Cut in half twice, then remove the cores and the seeds. Thinly slice into the water with vitamin C powder. Allow to stand for 15 minutes to prevent discoloration. In your blender, combine the lemon juice, spice and honey with half of the apple slices. Run the blender to mix, adding balance of apples and mixing until all has been blended to as smooth a sauce as desired. Chill before serving.

Main courses

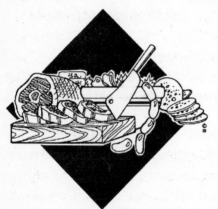

BAKED LENTILS WITH HONEY
2 C. lentils
1/2 lb. turkey sausage
4 cloves garlic, minced
1/4 C. finely chopped chutney
1/2 tsp. salt
1 tsp. prepared mustard
1/2 C. honey
Cook the lentils in a large pan with 4 cups of cold water. When they come to a boil, lower the heat to simmer and cook with a lid on for 1 hour. Drain off any liquid that is left. Meanwhile, fry the sausage, discarding any grease. Preheat the oven. Into the lentils, stir together the sausage, garlic, salt, mustard, and 1 cup of water. Empty out into a 2-quart shallow baking dish. Drizzle the honey over the top. Cover and bake at 325 degrees for 20 minutes. Remove cover and bake 20 minutes more.

OVEN FRIED CHICKEN WITH HONEY BUTTER SAUCE
1 broiler-fryer, cut up
1 c. whole wheat flour
2 t. salt
1/4 t. pepper
2 t. paprika
3 T. melted butter

Combine flour, salt, pepper, and paprika. Dip chicken pieces in mixture. Melt butter and roll chicken in butter. Lay in single layer, skin side up. Bake in 375 degree oven for 30 minutes. Turn chicken. Pour honey-butter sauce over top and finish baking.

Honey-Butter sauce:
To melted butter, add:
1/4 c. honey
1/4 c. lemon juice

Pour honey sauce over and bake another 30 minutes or until tender. Baste occasionally with sauce.

BAKED HAM WITH ORANGE HONEY SAUCE
1 (6 to 10 lb.) ham
Whole cloves
1 (6 oz.) can frozen orange juice, thawed
1 3/4 c. water
1/2 c. honey
1 t. dry mustard
1/2 t. salt
1 cinnamon stick
1/8 t. nutmeg
3 T. cornstarch

2 oranges, sectioned

Score ham; stud with cloves. Bake in moderate oven, 350 degrees, for 10 to 15 minutes per pound. While ham is baking, put undiluted orange concentrate, water, honey, dry mustard, salt, cinnamon stick, and nutmeg in a saucepan. Blend cornstarch with 1/4 cup of the mixture and return to saucepan. Cook over medium heat, stirring constantly, until mixture thickens and comes to a boil. Boil 1 minute. Remove from heat; cool. Brush ham with small amounts of sauce 2 or 3 times during last 30 minutes of baking time. Add orange slices to remaining sauce. Heat. Serve with ham.

MARINADE FOR HAM
1 c. catsup
1/4 c. light flavored honey
1/4 c. prepared mustard

Stir together and baste ham during last 30 minutes of baking.

EASY DINNER
2 T. oil
1 small onion, chopped
1 green pepper, chopped
1 glove garlic, minced
1 lb. ground beef
1 T. honey
2 t. salt
1 t. chili powder
1/4 lb. dry whole grain noodles
3 1/2 c. tomatoes
1 c. diced sharp Cheddar cheese

Heat oil in skillet. Add onion, pepper, garlic, and meat. Brown lightly, stirring constantly. When browned, drain excess oil and stir in honey, salt and chili powder. Blend well. Add noodles, tomatoes and cheese. Cover. Bring to steaming temperature; turn heat to low and continue cooking for 30 minutes or until noodles are done. Serves 6.

SPAGHETTI SAUCE
1/2 green pepper, chopped fine
2 cloves garlic, chopped fine
1 large onion, chopped fine
1/4 c. parsley, chopped fine
1/4 c. celery, chopped fine

Sauté in 1 tablespoon of oil until tender. Add 1 1/2 pounds ground beef. Brown lightly. Drain off liquid.
Add:
1 (No. 2) can tomatoes
1 (15 oz.) can tomato paste (or sauce)
2 T. honey
1/4 t. oregano
1/8 t. red pepper
Salt and pepper to taste
Sliced mushrooms (optional)

Cook for 2 hours on a low heat.

BARBECUED BEEF
1/3 C. honey
1/2 C. catsup
1/4 C. apple cider vinegar
2 tsp. Worcestershire sauce
1/4 tsp. maple extract

2 C. finely sliced roast beef (already cooked)

Using a large skillet, stir the honey together with the catsup, apple cider vinegar, Worcestershire sauce and maple extract. Simmer until thoroughly heated. Add the sliced roast beef and heat on simmer until steaming hot. Serve as barbecued beef sandwiches or as a main dish on top of steaming hot rice.

HOT HONEYED HALIBUT STEAK
2 halibut steaks
1 T. oil
2 T. honey
4 or 5 drops hot pepper sauce

Place the oil in a skillet and quickly saute the fish about 3 minutes on each side, turning only once. During the last minute of cooking, drizzle the honey-hot sauce mixture on the fish. Serve immediately.

MIXED BEAN CASSEROLE
one 2 1/2 lb. can baked beans (without tomato sauce)
one 2 1/2 lb. can red kidney beans, drained
one 2 1/2 lb. can green lima beans, drained
1/2 c. chopped onion
1/4 c. wine vinegar
1/4 c. chopped turkey bacon
1/4 c. water
1/4 c. honey
1 t. dry mustard
1 t. salt
1/2 c. chili sauce (or catsup)

Pepper to taste

In a large greased casserole, mix all ingredients. Bake at 300 degrees for 2 hours. Stir after first hour to mix well.

SWEET SOUR SAUCE
2 T. vinegar
1/4 c. honey
2 T. lemon juice
1 T. chopped pimento
1/8 t. paprika

Combine all ingredients and heat. Makes 2/3 cup.

Breakfast

HONEY BUTTER
2 parts honey
1 part butter

Let butter stand in room temperature until it is soft. Add honey and stir until well blended. Place in a tightly covered jar and place in refrigerator.

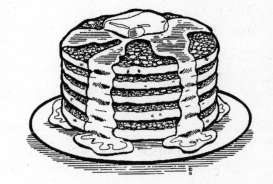

APPLE TOPPING
1 T. cornstarch
1 C. apple juice
1 1/2 T. honey
1 lg. apple, diced

Place all the ingredients in a medium saucepan and cook over medium heat, stirring constantly, until the sauce boils. Serve on waffles or pancakes.

BRAN DATE MUFFINS
1 C. whole wheat pastry flour
2 tsp. baking soda
1 1/4 C. wheat bran
1/2 C. chopped dates or raisins
1/2 C. honey
2 T. butter, softened to room temperature
2 eggs, well beaten
3/4 C. milk

In a large-sized mixing bowl, combine the dry ingredients. Stir in the chopped dates. Set aside. In another medium-sized mixing bowl, cream the honey and butter together until smooth. Add the eggs and beat until well blended. Next, add the milk and continue beating until smooth. Make a well in the center of the dry mixture and add the honey batter. Stir only until the dry ingredients are moistened. Spoon into 12 greased muffin pans. Bake in a preheated 350 degree oven for 20 to 25 minutes.

APPLE MUESLI
3 T. uncooked oatmeal
3 T. raisins
1 C. cold water
3 T. chopped walnuts
2 T. lemon juice
2 T. honey

1 lg. apple, unpeeled

Soak the oatmeal and raisins overnight in about 1 cup of cold water. The next morning, drain the water off. Stir in the chopped walnuts with the softened oatmeal and raisins. Add the lemon and honey which has been well blended. Grate the apple into the Muesli. Stir until evenly mixed.

PEAR AND OAT BRAN SCONES

1 C. whole wheat flour
1 tsp. baking soda
1 tsp. cream of tartar
1 tsp. cinnamon
1/3 C. butter
1 C. oat bran
1/3 C. currants or chopped raisins
3/4 C. diced fresh pear
2 egg whites
2 T. apple juice
2 T. honey
1 tsp. vanilla

Stir the first 4 ingredients together in a mixing bowl. Cut in the butter until the mixture resembles coarse crumbs. Stir in the oat bran, currants, and pear. Mix the egg whites, apple juice, honey and vanilla in another small bowl. Add to the dry ingredients, stirring only until moistened. The dough might seem a little sticky. Use a nonstick baking sheet or a lightly oiled baking sheet. Flour your hands and divide the dough into 8 balls. Flatten slightly. Drizzle just a touch of honey on the top of each sconce. Bake in a 400 degree oven for 10 to 12 minutes, until golden around the edges. Serve warm.

TROPICAL BREAKFAST BARS
2 C. dry rolled oats
1 C. whole wheat flour
1 C. oat flour
1 C. chopped dates
1/2 C. chopped, dried pineapple
1/2 C. chopped, dried papaya
1/3 C. sesame seeds
1/3 C. coconut
1 T. oil
1 T. honey
1 1/2 C. water
2/3 C. walnuts

Measure out and stir together the first 8 ingredients in a large mixing bowl. Place the walnuts, water, oil and honey in a blender and process until smooth. Add to the fruit mixture, stirring until well mixed. Press the mixture into a lightly greased 10" x 15" baking pan. Bake at 400 degrees for about 25 minutes. Cool slightly, then cut into 2" squares.

Breads

WHOLE WHEAT SESAME CRACKERS
2 C. whole wheat flour
2 tsp. baking powder
1 tsp. baking soda
1/2 tsp. cream of tarter
1/2 tsp. salt
3 T. honey
1/2 C. butter
3/4 C. buttermilk
1/4 C. sesame seeds

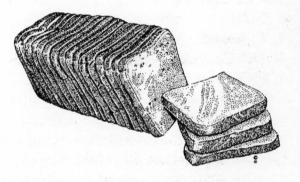

Stir the dry ingredients together in a large bowl. Add the honey and butter and cut in until the mixture looks like coarse crumbs. Make a well in the mixture and pour in the buttermilk, stirring only until moistened. Turn the dough out onto a well floured surface. Flour your rolling pin too. Then roll out to about 1/8" thick and cut with a biscuit cutter or a soup can. Place on ungreased baking sheets; prick with a fork and then sprinkle with sesame seeds. Bake in a preheated 350 degree oven for about 15 minutes or until lightly browned. If you like them crispy, place in a 200 degree oven, then turn oven off and leave them overnight. Remove and store in airtight containers.

WHOLE WHEAT BREAD
Mix:
1 T. honey
1/2 c. warm water
1 1/2 pkg. dry yeast
Set aside.
Mix and cook the following until thick and smooth:
1 c. whole wheat flour
1 1/2 c. water
Stir constantly; put in large bowl. Add to cooked flour in order, mixing well:
1/3 c. honey
1/3 c. powdered milk
1 scant t. salt
1/3 c. canola oil
1 egg
1 c. whole wheat flour
Add yeast mixture. Gradually add approximately 4 cups whole wheat flour and mix well. Let rise 1 hour; knead 3 minutes. Let rest 15 minutes; knead a few strokes and divide into 8 equal pieces. Braid into loaves; let rise until double and bake at 375 degrees for 30 to 35 minutes.

SWEET ROLLS
1 c. milk
1/4 c. honey
1/4 c. butter
1 t. salt
1 cake compressed yeast

1/2 c. lukewarm water
2 eggs
4 1/2 to 5 c. whole wheat flour
Scald milk. Add honey, butter and salt.
Soften yeast in lukewarm water and add to milk
mixture. Add beaten eggs and half the flour; beat
well. Butter hands and knead on a lightly floured
board until smooth. Place in a slightly greased
bowl. Cover and let rise in a warm place to double
in size. Punch down and form into rolls. Let rise
again about 1 hour. Bake at 400 degrees for 20 to
25 minutes.

HONEY CORN BREAD
1 c. sifted whole wheat flour
3 t. baking powder
1 t. salt
1 c. yellow corn meal
1 egg. slightly beaten
1 c. milk
1/4 c. melted butter
3 T. honey
Mix flour, baking powder and salt. Add corn
meal. Combine egg, milk, butter, and honey. Pour
into flour mixture and stir until just moistened.
Pour into buttered pan; bake in 425 degree oven
for about 20 minutes.

HONEY BLUEBERRY MUFFINS
1 c. whole wheat flour
1 c. barley flour
1 t. salt
3 t. baking powder

1 c. milk
4 T. honey
1 egg, beaten
1/4 c. melted butter
1/2 c. blueberries
    Sift flours with salt and baking powder. Mix
milk, honey, beaten egg, blueberries, and melted
butter. Add to dry ingredients. Stir quickly, just
long enough to moisten dry ingredients. Fill
greased muffin pans 1/2 full. Bake in a 350 degree
oven, for 35 minutes or until browned. Makes 12
muffins.

Desserts

HONEY FUDGE CAKE
3 (1 oz.) sq. unsweetened melted chocolate
1/3 c. milk
1/3 c. honey
1 egg, well beaten
1/2 c. butter
2/3 c. milk
1 1/4 t. vanilla
1 c. honey
2 eggs
2 c. sifted whole
wheat cake flour
1 t. baking powder
1/2 t. salt

    Combine melted chocolate, 1/3 cup milk, 1/3
cup honey and well beaten egg in saucepan. Cook
over low heat, stirring constantly, until thickened.
Cool. Cream butter and vanilla. Add 1 cup honey in

a fine stream, creaming until light and fluffy. Add remaining eggs, one at a time, beating well after each addition. Sift together flour, baking soda, baking powder, and salt. Combine cooled chocolate with 2/3 cup milk. Add dry ingredients to creamed mixture. Beat after each addition until smooth. Bake in 2 greased paper lined 9 inch round pans at 350 degrees for 25 to 30 minutes. Cool 5 minutes before removing from pan.

ICING
1/2 c. honey
1/4 c. pineapple juice or orange juice
   Bring juice and honey to quick boil. Cool; use pastry brush and apply to warm cake.

CREAM CHEESE FROSTING
8 oz. no-fat cream cheese
1/3 c. honey
1 t. vanilla
   Cream all ingredients until smooth.

HONEY CHOCOLATE SAUCE
one 6 oz. pkg. semi-sweet chocolate pieces
1/2 c. honey
3/4 c. evaporated milk
   Melt chocolate in honey over low heat. Stir to keep well blended. Add evaporated milk and stir until well blended. Cool.

CAROB-CHIP ZUCCHINI CAKE
1/2 C. butter, softened
1/4 C. canola oil

1 C. honey
2 eggs
1 tsp. vanilla
1/2 C. milk with 1 tsp. vinegar added
1 C. whole wheat flour
1 1/2 C. white flour
1/4 C. carob powder (or cocoa)
1/2 tsp. baking powder
1 tsp. baking soda
1/2 tsp. cinnamon
1/2 tsp. cloves
2 C. shredded zucchini
1/4 C. carob chips

In a large mixing bowl, cream together the butter with the oil, honey, eggs and vanilla, beating until light and fluffy. Add the milk and mix well. In a separate bowl, mix the dry ingredients. Stir the dry ingredients into the honey mixture, then mix with an electric mixer for 2 minutes. Stir in the zucchini. Place batter into a greased and floured 9 x 13" baking pan. Sprinkle the batter with carob chips. Bake in a 325 degree oven for 40 to 45 minutes or until done.

HONEY APPLE PIE
Pastry for double crust
6 apples
1 T. butter
2 T. lemon juice
1/2 t. cinnamon
1/2 c. honey

Line pie pan with pastry; roll thin and prick with fork. Pare fruit and slice thin. Arrange on pastry. Sprinkle the honey, lemon juice and cinnamon on top. Dot with bits of butter. Cover with perforated top crust. Press together at edges. Bake in a 450 degree oven, for 10 minutes. Reduce heat to 350 degrees and bake 25 to 30 minutes longer or until crust is slightly browned and the fruit is soft.

PUMPKIN PIE FILLING
1 (9 inch) unbaked whole wheat pastry shell
3/4 c. honey
3/4 c. nonfat dry milk solids
1/2 t. salt
1/2 t. cinnamon
1/2 t. mace
1/4 t. cloves
1 1/2 c. cooked pumpkin
2 eggs, well beaten
1 1/2 c. water
2 T. melted butter
1/2 t. ginger
 Mix dry ingredients well. Add other ingredients. Blend thoroughly. Turn into pastry shell. Bake 15 minutes at 425 degrees in preheated oven. Reduce to 350 degrees and bake 40 minutes longer.

PEANUT BUTTER SATIN PIE
1/2 C. peanut butter
1/2 C. butter, softened to room temperature
1/4 C. honey
1/4 C. non-instant powdered milk
1/2 lb. tofu

Cream the peanut butter together with the softened butter. Slowly add the honey, beating constantly. Stir in the powdered milk. Divide the tofu in 4 equal-sized pieces and add 1 at a time, beating well after each addition. Empty into a cooked pie shell. Chill until firmly set.

CAROB COOKIES
3/4 C. soft butter
1/2 C. honey
1 tsp. vanilla
1/2 tsp. salt
1 C. carob chips
1/2 C. chopped walnuts
1 C. whole wheat flour
1 C. white flour
1 C. dry oatmeal

Cream the softened butter and honey together. Add vanilla, salt and stir. In a separate bowl, measure out the flours, oatmeal, carob chips and nuts; mix together and add to the honey mixture, stirring together until blended. Roll in small balls and place on an ungreased cookie sheet. Flatten each ball with the prongs of a fork. Bake in a 325 degree oven for 15 minutes or until a light golden brown

HONEY PUMPKIN DROPS
1/2 C. butter, softened
1 C. honey
2 eggs, beaten
1 C. cooked mashed pumpkin
1 C. white flour

1 and 1/2 C. whole wheat flour
1/4 C. dry milk
1 T. baking soda
1 tsp. salt
2 tsp. cinnamon
1/2 tsp. nutmeg
1/4 tsp. ginger
1 C. chopped dates
1 C. chopped nuts

Cream the butter and honey together in a mixing bowl, until light and fluffy. Add the eggs and pumpkin; mix well. Mix all the dry ingredients in a small bowl. Add the dry ingredients to the honey mixture and stir until blended. Stir in the chopped dates and nuts. Drop by heaping teaspoonfuls onto a greased cookie sheet. Bake in the upper half of your oven at 350 degrees for 15 minutes. Remove from cookie sheet and cool on paper towels.

HONEY OATMEAL CHEWS
1/2 c. butter
3/4 c. honey
1 egg
1 t. vanilla
2/3 c. sifted whole wheat flour
1/2 t. baking soda
1/2 t. baking powder
1/4 t. salt
1 c. quick cooking rolled oats
1 c. flaked coconut
1/2 c. chopped almonds

Cream butter and honey until light and fluffy. Add egg and vanilla; beat well. Sift together flour, soda, baking powder, and salt. Add to creamed mixture. Stir in oatmeal, coconut and nuts. Spread in a greased 13 1/2 x 9 inch baking pan. Bake at 350 degrees for 20 to 25 minutes. When cool, cut into bars about 1 1/2 x 2 1/2 inches. Makes 30.

HONEY APPLESAUCE COOKIES
3 c. sifted whole wheat pastry flour
3/4 t. baking powder
1 1/4 t. salt
1/2 t. soda
1 t. cinnamon
1/4 t. cloves
3/4 c. butter
1 t. grated lemon rind
2 eggs (unbeaten)
1/2 c. honey
3/4 c. applesauce
3/4 c. coarsely chopped nuts
1 c. raisins

Measure sifted flour; add baking powder, salt and spices and sift again. Cream butter with lemon rind. Add eggs and honey; beat well. Add flour alternately with applesauce, a small amount at a time, beating after each addition until smooth. Mix in nuts and raisins. Drop by teaspoonfuls onto greased baking sheet. Bake in 400 degree oven for about 12 minutes.

HONEY NUT BROWNIES
1/4 c. butter

2 oz. chocolate
3/4 c. honey
2 eggs, well beaten
1/2 c. whole wheat flour
1/4 t. baking powder
1 t. vanilla
1 c. chopped walnuts

Melt chocolate and butter together. Mix in honey, then eggs. Sift together flour and baking powder. Combine with chocolate mixture. Add vanilla and nuts. Bake in a 7x11 inch well greased pan for 45 minutes at 300 degrees.

Jam & Jellies

CREAMED APRICOT JAM
1/2 lb. dried apricots
Water
1/2 C. creamed honey

Place the dried apricots in a bowl and cover with cold water. Allow to soak from 4 to 6 hours or until the water has been absorbed. When the dried apricots are soft but hold their shape, they are ready. Cut up enough apricots in very small pieces to make 1/3 cup; set aside. Grind the rest in your blender; making the apricots into a puree. Stir the creamed honey together with the apricot puree and the 1/3 cup of finely chopped apricots. No cooking is required.

HONEY CHUTNEY
2 qt. sour apples
2 green peppers

1/3 c. onions
3/4 lb. seedless raisins
1/2 T. salt
1 c. honey
Juice of 2 lemons and grated rind of 1 lemon
1 1/2 c. vinegar
3/4 c. tart fruit juice
3/4 T. ginger
1/4 t. cayenne pepper

Wash and chop fruit and vegetables. Add all other ingredients and simmer until thick like chili sauce.

Chapter 4

📖

GARLIC FACTS & REMEDIES
superherb from Mt. Olympus

"Gilroy, California is the only town in America where you can marinate a steak by hanging it on the clothesline." Will Rogers, regarding the "garlic capital" of America

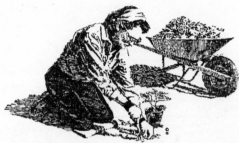

❀ PERSONAL PROFILE. A.F. was a young woman in her thirties who had just learned that she had advanced breast cancer. She had 2 young children at home and was not prepared for the doctor's warning: "Unless you undergo radical surgery, with chemotherapy and radiation therapy, you will probably die with a year." What could she do? She followed her doctor's advice. The therapy did not slow the cancer, which now appeared throughout her body, including her spine. "We are going to try a last ditch effort to save you with a radical procedure called bone marrow transplant" her doctor's told her. That also was ineffective at slowing the cancer. After 2 years of valiantly fighting cancer with every trick in the medical book, AF was told to "get her affairs in order".

She was not a quitter and certainly couldn't see someone else raising her kids, so she gathered all the information she could find on therapies for cancer that would strengthen her body's natural defense mechanisms. She changed her diet, dropping all animal food like beef and cheese. She went on a serious detoxification program to rid her body of accumulated toxins which drag down the immune system. She changed her way of thinking, eliminating negative thoughts and stressful events. She started taking supplements, including garlic extract. Within 6 weeks, the cancer was gone from her soft and hard tissue--even the bones showed no signs of cancer. What modern medicine could not do, Nature's simple healing agents could do. AF learned a very important lesson in healing: In order to reverse a disease, you must first change the underlying causes of the disease. Drugs and surgery can be temporarily helpful, but do not cure any disease. Only you can do that. In AF's case, garlic helped her to beat end stage terminal cancer.

If a human had invented garlic, then he or she would have surely been awarded the Nobel prize in medicine, plus given a cushy job at some prestigious university and retired handsomely on the dividends from the drug patent. But since humble Nature created garlic, you can buy it for pennies without prescription and with a list of therapeutic benefits that literally staggers the imagination.

Riddle me this: What drug can:
-lower fats in the blood to prevent heart disease
-thin out the blood to prevent strokes
-improve immune functions to fight infections and cancer
-regulate blood pressure
-regulate blood sugar levels
-energize
-detoxify the body
-and more

All while costing pennies a day with no side effects? Answer: No drug or even collection of drugs can do that. But garlic can.

A LONG AND HEROIC PAST

First mentioned about 6000 years ago, garlic, or allium sativum, has been a major player in human history. In the tomb of the Egyptian king, Tutankhamen, were found gold ornaments and 6 garlic bulb that were dried and perfectly preserved, about 3300 years after being placed there. Slaves who built the Great Pyramids relied heavily on the energizing power of garlic for their work, with unprecedented work strikes if the garlic supplies ran out.

As the Israelites wandered the desert after their exodus from Egypt, they longed for their meals with garlic: "Think of the fish we used to eat free in Egypt, the cucumbers, melons, leeks, onions, and garlic." (Numbers 11:4). Garlic was a major commodity of international trade, like we buy and sell wheat and soybeans. In Babylon around 538 BC, mention was made of a sale of garlic involving 15 million bulbs!! Romans and Greeks valued garlic for the strength it provided.

Hippocrates, father of modern medicine, used garlic and opium as common healers for infections and pain killing during primitive surgical amputations. Though garlic has been used for at least 4000 years as a primary healing agent, only recently have skeptics dropped their sarcasm as over 2000 scientific research articles now point toward the near-miraculous healing powers of this humble little vegetable.

Why did we reject a time-tested healing agent? From around 1800 to 1980, modern medicine was trying to "grow up" and detach itself from its roots, not unlike a troublesome teenager pushes away from its parent. In 1870, the medical journal Practitioner listed garlic as "a quaint and absurd medicament, now obselete among physicians." As of the First World Congress on Garlic, held in Washington, DC in 1990, garlic has been promoted to a first class, scientifically supported healing herb. Modern medicine is beginning to re-visit the many herbal preparations that allowed humanity to survive a couple of million years without the use of prescription drugs.

During the Black Plague of the 14th century in which 75 million people died throughout Europe, folks who ate and wore garlic were less likely to become infected. Thus, thieves would cloak themselves in garlic and rob the dead and the dying from plague-infested areas, giving birth to the infamous recipe for "Four Thieves vinegar and garlic". Since no one in those days knew anything about infectious organisms that cause plagues, it was assumed that garlic protected people from evil in general. And garlic does have an amazing cleansing ability. It gets rid of fleas on pets, worms from children's guts, bacteria from the blood, fat out of the body, toxins from the liver and generally purges bad things out of the good. For this reason, garlic developed a legendary ability to protect primitive people from evil, such as vampires and the "evil eye".

While garlic probably was originally cultivated somewhere in Asia, near Mongolia, and was spread around the world through traders, once garlic reached England it found great disfavor.

Royalty considered garlic a peasant's vegetable which quickly allowed people to smell the difference between paupers and princes. Even William Shakespeare (1564-1616) took a few cheap shots at garlic: "...eat no onions or garlic, for we are to utter sweet breath." (Midsummer's Night Dream). In Pearl Buck's Pulitzer Prize winning novel, The Good Earth, she speaks of the unmistakable smell of garlic on the breath of Chinese peasants.

Throughout all of these highs and lows, garlic went about its healing ways, unaffected by the pompous scorn of royalty and scientists. Throughout World Wars I and II, many combat physicians lacking sulfa drugs or antibiotics would praise the effectiveness of dressing wounds and treating infections with garlic. Garlic eventually became affectionately known as Russian or Chinese "penicillin".

American doctors were unimpressed by thousands of years of folk legends or even well-controlled scientific studies from other countries. No scientist in America wanted to be the first person to risk being ostracized by studying garlic. David Kritchevsky, a young post-doctoral student from the U.S., was studying in Switzerland. Dr. Kritchevsky's landlady was a vibrant woman of 66, who looked 44 and acted 22. Kritchevsky asked her secret to her youthful energy and she replied "a clove of garlic with each evening meal". As Kritchevsky probed this issue, he found more European data available on the scientific value of garlic, which had been overlooked in America. Kritchevsky was the first credible scientist in the

U.S. to study garlic, but we can credit his zesty landlady with triggering the academic curiosity.

WHO EATS IT?

World lovers of the "lowly stinking rose" know garlic in Mexico as "ajo", as "knofloock" in Holland, as "niniku" in Japan, and as "chesnok" in Moscow. The United Nations Food and Agriculture Organization lists the world's consumption of garlic at about 5 billion pounds (2.3 billion kg), or roughly a half a clove of garlic per day per person. China, India, Spain, South Korea, Thailand, and Egypt respectively are the world's dominant producers of garlic.

In the past 25 years, garlic production has quadrupled in the U.S. Ninety percent of the garlic consumed in the U.S. is grown within a 90 mile radius of Gilroy, California. If you are a true garlic fan, then this town is "Mecca". Each summer in Gilroy, 150,000 "true believers" in garlic make their pilgrimage to belly up to restaurants to eat garlic ice cream, garlic beer, and garlic pie as Gilroy celebrates cornering the market on this $55 million dollar annual industry which is growing rapidly in America.

There are somewhere between 30 and 300 different strains of garlic grown around the world, from the intense heat of the Sahara desert, to the rain-soaked tropics, to the wind-swept northern prairies. Few plants are as tenacious and adaptable as garlic. My wife, Noreen, and myself had an interesting experience with last summer's garden. No one in our vicinity had much luck with their vegetable garden, including us. We mowed the garden in September and began planning on better luck next year. The day before Christmas, after several days of 10 degree F. weather, little rain for the past 4 months, and absolutely no tending to the garden, we found a row of garlic plants vigorously popping through the other vegetation. We had fresh garlic from our garden for that Christmas dinner.

One of the reasons for garlic's extraordinary popularity throughout human history is that it will grow almost anywhere, almost anytime of the year, in almost any soil, with very little tending, and will defend surrounding plants from insects while its at it.

WHAT'S IN IT?

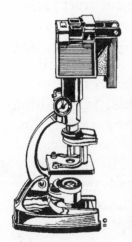

"The deeper you look into garlic's wonderful chemistry, the more you tend to discover what you didn't know before." Dr. Eric Block, professor of the State University of New York, at the First World Congress on Garlic

If you have seen the movie "Medicine Man" with Sean Connery, then you can get a feel for the complexities of finding the "active ingredient". In this movie, Connery is a physician in the Amazon Jungle who feels that he has found the cure for cancer, but cannot quite re-create his initially successful herbal formula. As he races to find the "active ingredient", the jungle is rapidly being consumed by bulldozers and fire. Finally, he finds that the active ingredient: the feces from spiders after they had eaten out of the sugar bowl.

The reason for this little anecdote is to prepare you for the complexities and confusion surrounding the "active ingredients" that are to be credited for garlic's amazing healing powers. You see, the health care industry in America is built around our $80 billion per year drug business. In spite of pressure from Congress to lower drug prices and world wide recessions in the health care arena, international pharmaceutical companies still report 20-30% annual profit margins to their stock holders. Drugs are profitable because they are patented and therefore protected from competition by law and therefore can extract major profits from those who need the drugs. Drug companies feel that they have a right to recoup their $150 million investment that is required to jump through the 5 years worth of hoops setup by the Food and Drug Administration for official FDA approval.

Garlic cannot be patented because it is a natural product. But if someone can find the active ingredient in garlic, then perhaps a major drug company can create a synthetic analog, or chemical that is similar in structure, and then someone can make a serious fortune off the healing actions of garlic. That is why this quest for the "holy grail" of the active ingredient in garlic.

Meanwhile, according to a nutrient content chart from the United States Department of

Agriculture, here is what's in 100 grams (about 3.5 ounces) of edible garlic:

NUTRIENT CONTENT	
Water	61.3%
Carbohydrate	30.8 g
Protein	6.2 g
Fiber	1.5 g
Fat	0.2 g
Ash	1.5 g
Potassium	259 mg
Phosphorus	202 mg
Calcium	29 mg
Sodium	19 mg
Iron	1.5 mg
Ascorbic acid	15 mg
Niacin	0.5 mg
Thiamine	0.25 mg
Riboflavin	0.08 mg
Vitamin A	trace

This nutrient listing is very unremarkable, but it is like a cover-story for Superman--a bland appearance belies the dynamo within. Let's glean from the world's best scientists and look behind the scenes at the REAL active ingredients in garlic.

•PROTEIN. While garlic is only a modest 6% protein, the unique sulfur-bearing amino acids in garlic provide a piece of the puzzle in deciphering its potent healing ability. S-allyl cysteine, S-allyl mercaptocysteine, S-allyl methyl cysteine, and gamma glutamyl S-allyl cysteine are among the unique amino acids found in garlic that are primary candidates for potent medicines. One of these agents, S-allyl cysteine, is odorless, stable, and safe and has been demonstrated by itself to reduce cholesterol in the blood, thin out the blood to prevent strokes, prevent cancer in animals, and detoxify the liver.

•ENZYMES. Enzymes are the chemical "workers" that take things apart and put things together. Garlic contains at least 9 water-soluble enzymes. One of the more important enzymes, alliinase, acts on alliin to produce allicin, which was once considered the "active ingredient" in garlic. However, allicin is unstable and deteriorates within a few hours. Something else in garlic will have to get credit for the incredible health-restoring abilities.

•CARBOHYDRATES. Most of garlic is a collection of starches and sugars. There are 17 identified sugars, including fructo-oligosaccharides (FOS) which help to promote the growth of friendly bacteria (like acidophilus) in the gut. FOS is another reason why garlic helps so many people with so many different health problems.

•VITAMINS, MINERALS. Based on what we know, there is nothing special here.

•TRACE MINERALS. There is a small amount of selenium in garlic which could help explain its ability to detoxify the body and protect against the ravages of aging. Also, garlic contains 1 part per billion of germanium, which is not much unless your body is starving for this mysterious trace mineral that seems to help oxygenate the cells.

•NUCLEOSIDES. These are substances that help to build the DNA in the body, which is the blueprints to make a whole new you. There are six different nucleosides in garlic, including adenosine, which may be another clue to garlic's value.

•SPECIAL OILS. This is where the stinky part is found. Among the oily compounds in garlic are diallyl disulfide, diallyl trisulfide, and small amounts of other volatile and unstable oils.

Some of the experts claim that only aged and deodorized garlic has any health value. Some claim that raw garlic is actually harmful. Some claim to have a unique process for extracting their own favorite "active ingredient" from garlic. There's probably value in all of these variations on garlic. Excessive amounts of raw garlic (30 cloves per day) which were used during WWI and WWII to treat infections have been shown to create anemia, diarrhea, and other problems in some sensitive individuals.

✍ RECOMMENDATIONS. There is probably a combination of substances mentioned above and trace ingredients yet-to-be discovered that account for the miraculous and versatile healing powers of garlic. Let me offer some simple advice for using garlic:

1) Eat no more than 2 cloves of **raw** garlic each day

2) Eat roasted or cooked garlic regularly, with an average of 2 cloves or more daily.

3) Use pill concentrates of garlic IN ADDITION TO, not instead of whole garlic in the diet. The German FDA allows certain health claims to be

made on garlic products that contain a specified amount of allicin, which they feel to be the active ingredient. You may want to buy garlic supplements with a guaranteed amount of allicin. However, aged and deodorized garlic, Kyolic, has been used in many of the scientific studies which support garlic's healing power. Kyolic has little or no allicin content. More than coincidentally, there are numerous cultures around the world where the tradition is to harvest garlic in the fall, then wrap the garlic in herbal leaves (like basil) and store it for later use. This aged garlic would probably have heightened healing powers, based upon a great deal of scientific evidence available today.

WHAT CAN IT DO FOR US?
GARLIC REMEDIES

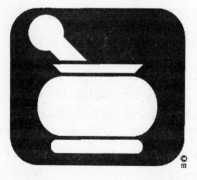

Prevents and reverses heart disease. By lowering the amounts of fats in the blood and reducing the body's own production of cholesterol in the liver, garlic should be a first choice for every cardiologist around the world. The "French paradox" is a puzzle in which the French people eat more fat, smoke more, and get little exercise, yet have about half the incidence of heart disease compared to Americans. Some experts attribute this puzzle to the French passion for red wine, which certainly has its merits. Yet other experts give more credit to the high amounts of garlic consumed by the French in saving them from an otherwise dismal fate of heart disease.

Garlic works on several levels to prevent and reverse heart disease:

1) by slowing the liver's own production of cholesterol

2) by mobilizing fat stores throughout the body into the bloodstream so the fat can be burned for energy or excreted.

In a review article of 18 different studies testing garlic in human heart disease patients and published in the British Journal of Clinical Pharmacology, garlic clearly lowered the "bad fats" (cholesterol, triglycerides, LDL) and raised the good fat (HDL). In a study from India, researchers divided 432 heart disease patients into 2 groups. One group received daily garlic supplements, while the other group did not. The group receiving garlic had a 30% reduction in repeat heart attacks in year 2 and a 60% reduction in year 3.

Reduces and stabilizes blood pressure. One of those sulfured amino acids in garlic is very effective at preventing angiotensin 1 from being converted into angiotensin 2, which provides you with the net benefit of lowering blood pressure. If you have low blood pressure, garlic will help to bring it up to normal, thus doing what no drug can do: bringing your body into optimal functioning regardless of what the problem is. In one study looking at 20 patients with high blood fats, 4 weeks of garlic therapy provided an average of 10% drop across the board in 1) blood fats, 2) blood pressure, 3) fibrinogen, or clotting activity.

Prevents and reverses stroke. By thinning the blood, garlic is able to prevent the deadly buildup of blood clots that choke off tiny capillaries to create strokes or the loss of function that is often associated with aging. We need to have our blood clot when our skin is penetrated, to avoid bleeding to death. Thromboxane helps us do this. Yet we don't want that clotting mechanism kicking in too soon, which creates sticky clumps of blood that get stuck in capillaries and cause stroke or a slow suffocating death throughout the body. Prostacyclin helps us do this. Garlic helps to keep the clotting mechanism in balance by inhibiting thromboxane, but not prostacyclin.

Fibrin is the web of clotting material that forms all too early in the bloodstream of many people. Fibrinogen is an accurate barometer of how much clotting is going on in the bloodstream. Researchers found that garlic lowered fibrinogen levels in adult men, even after being fed 3.5 ounces (100 grams) of butter, which normally really cranks up the clotting machinery. Researchers at George Washington University School of Medicine report that garlic inhibits blood clotting better than aspirin.

Fights infections and cancer. By stimulating the immune system to get more active at killing cancer cells and by helping the body to eliminate built up toxins, garlic can help us in our failing efforts in the "war on cancer." Scientists find that garlic is deadly to invading bacteria, virus, or tumor cells, but is harmless to normal healthy body cells; thus offering the hope of the truly "selective toxin" against cancer that is being sought worldwide. Your body's army of 20 trillion immune cells give up their lives to kill invaders and dispose of garbage throughout your body. When the immune system is overwhelmed; infections, cancer, and premature aging are the result. Garlic stimulates various components of the immune system into greater production and activity, including macrophages (literally: "big eaters"), and Natural Killer cells, which are the "Rambos" in your personal war on cancer.

Pasteur noted that garlic killed all of the bacteria in his petri dishes. Garlic has been found to stimulate natural protection against tumor cells. Garlic and onions fed to lab animals helped to decrease the number of skin tumors.[1] Mice with a genetic weakness toward cancer were fed raw garlic with a lower-than-expected tumor incidence.[2] Tarig Abdullah, MD of Florida found that white blood cells from garlic-fed people were able to kill 139% more tumor cells than white cells from non-garlic eaters.[3] Dr. Abdullah also used garlic extract in 7 AIDS patients with encouraging results: reduction of diarrhea and other symptoms with improvement in Natural Killer cell count and activity. Researchers are excited about the early encouraging results of incubating cancer cells in garlic, which disrupts their metabolism, then injecting this "vaccine" into a cancer patient.

In one area of China, the people eat an average of 7 cloves of cooked garlic each day. Their stomach cancer incidence is about 3 per 100,000. Yet in nearby Qixia County where garlic is rarely consumed, the stomach cancer incidence is 1300% higher, or 40 per 100,000. Stomach cancer is one of the more common cancers around the world.

Garlic has been shown to be effective in treating bacterial infections (both gram negative and positive), yeast infections (including Candida Albicans), viruses (including polio), and intestinal parasites of all sorts. To paraphrase a famous TV commercial: "Don't leave home without it."

Detoxification. While the 20th century has brought us many advances through technology, we are also drowning in our irresponsible dumping of our high tech waste products. Toxic burden in the air, food, and water supply is contributing to our immune disorders, including cancer, AIDS, arthritis, multiple sclerosis, chronic fatigue, and more. The unique sulfur bearing amino acids in garlic seem to be able to "cage" heavy metals, like lead and mercury, and carry them out of the body in a process called "chelation" (say: key-lay-shun). Additionally, something in garlic supercharges the liver to produce more of the vital enzyme, glutathione-S-transferase, for general detoxification of various chemicals.

Protect against pollution. Various agents in garlic have the ability to prevent known cancer-causing agents, like aflatoxin from moldy peanuts and DMBA from tobacco, from binding to the delicate DNA, which could then trigger cancer.

Blood sugar regulation. Attention diabetics and hypoglycemics: garlic may be able to improve your current condition. In animal studies done at the United States Department of Agriculture, researchers found that garlic helped the liver to pull sugar out of the blood and encouraged the pancreas to make more insulin. The net effect was to bring blood sugar to an ideal level. This benefit alone could account for much of garlic's anti-aging effect.

Weight loss. "Then I tried the garlic diet. You don't lose any weight, but no one will come near you. And from a distance, you look thinner." Robert Orben, famous comedian. All kidding aside. Garlic can help reduce unnecessary appetite cravings through its ability to regulate blood sugar. Garlic can also reduce the body's production of fats while mobilizing stubborn fat out of its hiding places throughout the body. And because garlic can elevate the rate at which we burn calories, basal metabolism, garlic is a must for anyone wanting to lose weight and/or fat stores, like body builders.

Asthma Fighter. Take 1 tsp of this tonic with water every 15 minutes until the spasm is controlled. Afterward, give the patient 1 tsp every two or three hours for the rest of the day. Recipe: Take 1/2 pound peeled garlic buds, add equal amounts vinegar and distilled water to cover the buds; 1/2 pint glycerin and 1 1/2 pounds of honey. Put peeled garlic, vinegar and water in a wide-mouthed jar, close tightly and shake well. Let it stand in a cool place for four or five days, shaking twice daily. Add the glycerin, shake the jar and let stand one more day. Strain and blend in the honey. Store in a cool place.

Tooth ache. For gum or tooth problems, mix up a poultice of crushed garlic in peanut butter and apply to the affected area.

Congestion. For colds, bronchitis, catarrh, coughs, and laryngitis; use garlic as fresh, garlic, lozenge, or pills.

Infections. For middle-ear infections, sore throats, sinusitis, tonsillitis, gum infections, and mouth ulcers.

Digestive system. For diarrhea, gastroenteritis, dysentery, colitis, food poisoning, constipation, indigestion, and hemorrhoids. For hemorrhoids insert a small wad of crushed garlic and vitamin E oil from a capsule into the rectum at bedtime.

Urinogenital. For candidiasis, cysitis, thrush, and vaginitis.

Skin. For abscesses, acne, athlete's foot, ringworm, yeast-like infection, suppurating wounds, and ulcers.

Circulation. For atherosclerosis, vascular thrombosis, high blood fat, high blood pressure, and high blood cholesterol.

Blood sugar regulation. For high blood sugar (type 2 diabetes, non-insulin dependent) and hypoglycemia.

Protection from bee stings, non-lethal bites, contaminants, poisoning from heavy metals, and hangovers.

Immune system. For bacterial & fungal infections, lice & ticks, and worms. Four Thieves'

Vinegar is supposedly what the thieves drank to prevent them getting the Black Plague. It is both antiseptic and very aromatic. Take 7 g (1/4 oz) each of calamus root, cinnamon, ground nutmeg, lavender, mint, rosemary, rue, sage and wormwood, and two minced heads of garlic. Add 2 pt of cider vinegar. Cover and keep warm for five days. Strain and add 7 g (1/4 oz) of powdered camphor before bottling.

Aphrodisiac. Pound garlic with fresh coriander and add to wine.

Winter tonic. Steep three or four crushed cloves of garlic in a small bottle of brandy in a dark cupboard for fourteen days. Sip a tablespoon several times each day. Such a tincture was recommended in the eighteenth century by Dr. James Lind (founder of the link between limes and scurvy) for seamen on cold winter journeys.

Energy Food from Siberia. Mince four heads of garlic and four fresh onions. Boil 8 oz of barley in 2 pt of water until all the liquid is gone; do the same with 8 oz of oats, then mince both grains. Mince 2 oz of dried valerian root. Combine all these with 2 lb of honey until it is like a thick cream. Spread it one inch thick and let it set for a day. Cut it into one inch squares. Take three to six a day.

Recovery Soup. There is nothing like this easy-to-prepare soup to get you back on your feet. Put 2 full teaspoons miso, 1-2 cloves crushed garlic, a little grated onion, and a squeeze of vinegar in a mug or bowl. Add boiling water or vegetable stock, and mix well. Add a dash of soy sauce to taste.

HOW TO PREPARE YOUR GARLIC REMEDIES

Pills. Preferably as Kyolic aged deodorized garlic. Other garlic supplements with allicin are also available at your health food store. Follow directions on the label of the product.

Fresh cooked cloves. Break up a bulb of garlic into its smaller cloves. Do not peel the cloves. Place cloves in a coffee cup. Sprinkle olive oil and some seasoning, such as Spike, over the cloves. Cover with plastic wrap and place cup in microwave for 40-60 seconds, depending on how many cloves and how large. The resulting product is tasty, somewhat deodorized, and still quite therapeutic. Take liberally before, during, and after cold. Eat 6 cloves daily as a preventive remedy.

Syrups. Put 250 g (8 oz) of minced or crushed garlic in a 1 or 2 pt wide-mouthed jar. Almost fill with equal parts of apple cider vinegar and distilled water. Cover and let stand in a warm place for four days, shaking a few times a day. Add 1 cup of glycerin and let stand for a day. Strain through a cloth, add 1 cup of honey, and stir thoroughly. Keep cool. For deep coughs, sore throats. chronic bronchitis, high blood pressure, and circulation problems, take 1 tablespoon three times a day with meals.

Simpler syrup. Pour 1 pt of boiling water over 60 g (2 oz) of minced or crushed garlic. Keep in a cool place for 10 hours. Strain, and add 1 tablespoonful of vinegar and enough honey to make a syrup. Sip 1 tablespoonful three times a day as an expectorant. To this can be added: 1) 15 g (or

1/2 oz) of grated horseradish. This encourages sweating and is good for bronchitis. 2) 15 g (1/2 oz) of bruised fennel and caraway seeds. This soothes digestive problems.

Tea and Gargle. Brew 2 tablespoons of dried sage and four or five minced or crushed cloves of garlic in 2 pt of boiling water. Cover and stand until lukewarm. Take 1 small teacupful four or five times a day and gargle every half hour. For tonsillitis and to reduce mucous.

Bug spray for your garden. Take 3 oz of chopped garlic and let soak in 2 tsp (50 cc) of mineral oil for 24 hours. Then slowly add a pint of water in which 1/4 oz of dish soap has been dissolved, and stir well. Strain liquid through fine gauze and store in china or glass container to prevent a reaction with metals. Use it in a dilution of one part solution to 20 parts of water to begin with, then one to 100 thereafter. Apply to plants as spray.

Inhalant. Take three or four cloves of minced or crushed garlic and a teaspoon of apple vinegar. Add 1 pt. of boiling water and inhale the fumes. For nasal congestion.

External Remedies

Infections. Apply crushed fresh garlic as close as possible to the site of the infection, provided care is taken to keep the surrounding area free from possible blistering and provided you are prepared to put up with some initial stinging. If it burns too much, let it stand for a few minutes and try again.

Poultice. To apply garlic to a small area, first put petroleum jelly on the skin around it to prevent blistering. Put a small amount of minced garlic onto a piece of gauze and tape it in place with adhesive tape. Leave it on for 15-30 minutes. For athlete's foot, abscesses, boils, and other skin infections.

Poultice. To treat and soothe a wider area, you can use this bread poultice. Finely grate 60 g (2 oz) of garlic and add a crumbled 450 g (1 lb) wheat meal loaf of bread soaked in cold milk. Apply to the skin.

Poultice. For treating acne, spots, and mouth ulcers, simply hold or rub a bruised clove against the place. Russians used to press a half walnut shell filled with crushed garlic to the skin as a means of getting it into the system.

Poultice. Mix equal parts of zinc-oxide ointment, lanolin, and freshly ground garlic. As always, use a glass or ceramic container, not a metal one. Store in a covered jar. For eczema and hemorrhoids.

Poultice for boils and swellings. Take garlic, chervil, radish, turnip, raven's foot, honey, and pepper. Pound the plants and boil them in honey.

Garlic in Oil. Mince or crush 250 g (8 oz) of garlic and put it in a wide jar. Add enough olive oil to cover the garlic. Close the jar tightly and shake a few times a day. Stand it in a warm place for three days, then strain through a cloth. Keep the mixture cool. For earaches, put a few drops, warmed, in the ear on some cotton wool. For aches, sprains, and minor skin disorders, rub on; heating may help ease the pain. You can also add essential oils such as eucalyptus, cypress, or myrrh to the oil.

Scalp cleanser. Mix together 10 tablespoons castor oil and ten cloves of minced garlic. Cover and leave for thirty-six hours then strain and bottle. Massage it into the hair and scalp and wrap the head in a warm towel. After an hour, shampoo the hair normally. Useful for removing head lice.

Hemorrhoid suppository. Scrape a clove to produce juice, insert it into the rectum, and leave overnight. Repeat as needed.

Heal the Garden. Garlic will help protect your plants as well as yourself and your pets. An insecticide formula: Soak thirty minced cloves of garlic in 2 teaspoons (10 ml) mineral oil for 24 hours. Dissolve 7 g (1/4 oz) of an oil-based soap in 1 pt of water and add it to the garlic, stirring thoroughly. Strain and store the liquid in a glass or ceramic container. Use it as a spray on your plants at a dilution of between 1 part in 20 and 1 part in 100 of water.

Insect Repellent. Take 1 cup of sunflower of sesame seed oil. 1/2 cup of fresh feverfew (Tanacetum parthenium) or tansy (Tanacetum vulgare) flowers, or 1 tablespoon of the dried flowers, and eight cloves of minced garlic. Simmer the oil and blossoms for 15 minutes, cool and add the garlic. Bottle the mixture and keep it for five days, shaking two or three times a day, then strain. It can also be used as a remedy for bites.

Gargle or made into lozenges:
4 ounces freshly-sliced garlic
1 pint raw apple cider vinegar

20 ounces honey
        Equipment:
1 quart saucepan
Cheesecloth
Large mixing bowl
Wooden spoon
Candy thermometer
Large strainer
Straining cloth
Rubber gloves
1 pint amber storage bottle
Label

Slice the garlic. Pour the vinegar in the saucepan, stir in the garlic and bring to a boil, then reduce heat and simmer for 5 minutes tightly covered. Strain and press out the garlic, using rubber gloves, then return the liquid to the pan and stir in the honey. Cook down, keep on medium high heat and uncovered until the mixture reaches the consistency of thick syrup. On a candy thermometer, the temperature should read approximately 200 degrees. At this point, you can decant the syrup into an amber glass jar. Use for sore throats or a "healthy" candy.

GARLIC BREATH

If your breath is too strong from eating garlic, chew some sprigs of parsley, mint caraway, fenugreek seeds, or take a long bath in very warm water and the garlic oils will evaporate. Use the first recipe in the next chapter for cooked garlic in the microwave, which has "tamed" much of the nasty flavor and odor. Or you can use any number

of odorless and tasteless garlic supplements on the
market today.

1. Belman, S., Carcinogenesis, vol.4, no.8, p.1063, 1983
2. Kroning, F., Acta Unio Intern. Contra. Cancrum, vol.20, no.3, p.855, 1964
3. Abdullah, TH, et al., Journal of the National Medical Association, vol.80, no.4, p.439, Apr.1988

Chapter 5

📖

GARLIC RECIPES
cooking with Nature's most potent herb

"Let food be your medicine and your medicine be your food." Hippocrates, father of modern medicine, circa 400 B.C.

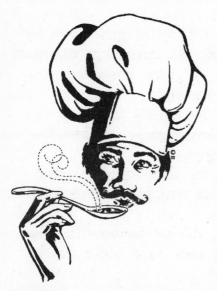

✿ PERSONAL PROFILE. JT was a bright professional in his 40s with a promising career ahead of him. He spoke of his enjoyment of his work and his love for his family. Yet he also was having problems with heart burn, or acid indigestion. Maybe the stress of his hectic schedule was getting to him. He was understandably concerned about taking drugs or even antacids on a regular basis to relieve his stomach problems. He asked me for help. I offered two simple suggestions that solved his problem. First, start each day with meditation or prayer. Get yourself into a relaxed state before the events of the day begin flying at you. Second, eat several bananas throughout the day and finish each day with a tablespoon of raw honey before bedtime. JT found almost instant relief and was able to continue his fulfilling and productive life without the risk of drugs to treat his upset stomach. Just another example of more simple solutions from Nature for complex modern health problems.

START OUT SLOW AND DEVELOP A TASTE FOR GARLIC

Now that you have learned all the healing benefits of eating garlic, this chapter will help you to incorporate more garlic into your diet. Start with the amounts below, which are on the low side. As your tastes change, you may wish to add more:

For meats: Use 1/8 to 1/4 tsp of garlic powder or two to three cloves of fresh garlic for every two pounds of meat.

Sauces: Use 1/8 to 1/4 tsp of garlic powder or two cloves of fresh garlic for three cups of sauce.

Soups: Add 1/8 tsp of garlic powder or two cloves of fresh garlic per serving.

Pickled foods: Add 1/8 to 1/4 tsp of dehydrated, chopped or minced garlic, or two to three fresh cloves per serving.

Relishes: Add 1/8 tsp dehydrated minced garlic or two fresh cloves to two pints of chutney or relish.

*When frying garlic, do not brown the herb because it will change the taste to a bitter flavor.

GARLIC EQUIVALENTS

Garlic usually comes as a "bulb" or "head" when buying fresh. Breaking the bulb into the sections will give you "cloves".

The following is a list of equivalents when replacing fresh garlic with garlic substitutes:

1/8 teaspoon garlic powder, or instant minced garlic or garlic chips = one average size clove of fresh garlic.

1/2 teaspoon of garlic salt is equivalent to one average size clove of fresh garlic.

General Recipes with Garlic

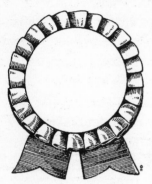

BLUE RIBBON GARLIC IN LESS THAN A MINUTE
1 head of garlic
1 Tbs olive oil
Spike seasoning
Break up the garlic head. Do not peel. Place in glass cup. Sprinkle oil and seasoning over the cloves. Cover with plastic wrap. Microwave for 45-55 seconds. Peel cloves. Taste like spring potatoes. Delicious!!

ROASTED GARLIC
10-12 large garlic cloves, peeled
2 Tbs butter
2 Tbs olive oil
Salt to taste
Pinch of white pepper
Preheat oven to 350 degrees. Heat the butter and olive oil in a oven proof casserole dish over medium heat. Add peeled cloves, side by side, and make sure they are well coated. Bake for 20 minutes, basting from time to time. Add salt and pepper. Serve as an appetizer with toast or as a vegetable side dish.

CHARCOAL ROASTED WHOLE GARLIC

Place whole bulbs of garlic, basted with oil, salt and pepper, directly in white hot but not flaming coals. When they're lightly browned, they're ready. Allow the bulbs to cool and break off the cloves.

Sauces and side dishes

SESAME SEED & GARBANZO DIP

1/2 cup crushed sesame seeds
16 ounces of cooked garbanzo beans, drained
4 cloves garlic
1/4 cup freshly squeezed lemon juice
2 tbsp fresh parsley

Combine the sesame seeds, beans, garlic and lemon juice in a food processor until smooth. Heat in a double boiler until sauce is heated through. Place in dip dish and garnish with parsley. Serve as a dip for vegetables and whole grain bread sticks.

ITALIAN PASTA SAUCE

2 quarts canned tomatoes
three 6-ounce cans tomato paste
1 green pepper, chopped
2 tbsp. each oregano and sweet basil
8 garlic cloves, minced
2 tsp. minced onion
1 bay leaf
2 tsp. honey
1 tsp. lime juice

Combine all of the ingredients in a large pan. Bring to a gentle simmer over medium heat. Let simmer at least one hour. The longer the sauce simmers, the better the flavor. When cooking is completed, remove the bay leaf. This sauce keeps for long periods in the freezer. Makes 2 1/2 quarts.

PESTO SAUCE
6 large garlic cloves
1 packed cup fresh parsley, tough stems removed
1 packed cup basil leaves, tough stems removed
1 cup olive oil
1/2 cup grated Parmesan cheese

Place the garlic, parsley, and basil in a blender and mix until all the ingredients are finely chopped. Then add the olive oil and blend for 20 seconds. Add the grated cheese and blend for another 15 seconds. This recipe makes about 1 1/2 cups. The extra sauce can be stored in the refrigerator for up to three weeks or kept in the freezer for about two months. Be sure that the basil leaves and parsley are submerged in the olive oil. Warm to room temperature before using.

MILD SALSA
dash of commercial hot pepper sauce
1 large tomato, chopped
1 medium avocado, chopped
1 tbsp. minced fresh cilantro
1 tbsp. fresh lime juice
4 cloves garlic, minced
1/2 tsp. salt

Combine all of the ingredients and mix well in a food processor. Yields about two cups of mild sauce.

GARLIC SPAGHETTI

Put spaghetti in boiling salted water. When spaghetti is half cooked, add three or four cloves of sliced, fried garlic, and 4 tablespoons olive oil, with pepper and salt. Finish cooking spaghetti. Drain and cover with grated cheese.

HUMMUS

1 can (15 ounces) of chickpeas, including liquid
1/4 cup tahini or sesame paste
2 tbsps. lemon juice
2 tbsps. lime juice
1 tbsp. orange juice
3 large garlic cloves, cut into thirds
1/2 tsp. cumin
Salt to taste
Chopped fresh parsley to garnish

Drain the chickpeas, reserving their liquid. Put them into a blender or food processor. Add the tahini, citrus juices, garlic, cumin, and 1/4 cup of chickpea liquid. Blend or process slowly, adding more chickpea liquid if required, until the entire mixture has become smooth. Season to taste with salt. Sprinkle with chopped parsley and serve with pita bread.

WILD RICE AND GARLIC

2 cloves fresh garlic, minced
1/2 cup chopped onion

2 tbsps. butter
14 ounces water
1 cup cooked wild rice
11 ounces homemade (or canned) cream of
mushroom soup
1/2 cup sliced green onions
1/4 cup sliced, almonds

Combine garlic and onion in a skillet, sautéing with butter until tender. Add rice, water and soup and heat in skillet until warm. Stir in green onions, cover and let simmer for ten minutes. Garnish with sliced almonds.

Vegetables with garlic

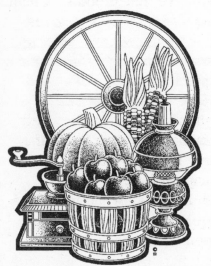

NO MEAT ROAST
2 eggs
3/4 cup milk
1/2 cup minced onion
2 cloves garlic, minced
2 cups ground walnuts or
pecans
2 cups whole wheat
bread crumbs
1/2 cup chopped celery
4 tsp butter
1/2 tsp powdered sage
1 tbsp chopped parsley

Pour 1/2 cup water in skillet and cook onion and garlic slowly for 5 minutes. Beat eggs well, adding milk, then add to remaining ingredients. Mix well and put in oiled baking dish. Cook 30 to 45 minutes, basting with equal parts hot water and melted butter.   Serve plain or with any desired gravy.

STUFFED MUSHROOMS WITH GARLIC & PARSLEY
12 large fresh mushrooms
1 tbsp. finely chopped lemon peel
1 tbsp. finely chopped lime peel
2 tbsps. fresh lemon juice
2 tbsps. fresh lime juice
Salt to taste
2 tbsps. olive oil
4 garlic cloves, finely chopped
1 cup chopped fresh parsley
6 tbsps. fresh bread crumbs

Remove the stems from the mushrooms. Clean the mushrooms.   Preheat the oven to 375 degrees. Arrange the mushrooms on a tray, concave side up, and lightly sprinkle each mushroom cap with lemon and lime juice and the chopped peels of both. Season with salt to taste.   Heat the oil in a skillet over a medium-high heat, then add the garlic, and sauté lightly about two minutes. Remove from the heat and add the parsley and bread crumbs.   Stir well.   Fill each mushroom cap with the filling mixture.   Arrange the filled mushrooms on an oiled cookie sheet, with the filling side turned up.   Bake for 15 minutes, the mushroom caps should stay firm.

EGGPLANT ANTIPASTO
4-6 eggplants
4 tomatoes, chopped
1 head of garlic, crushed or finely chopped

Fresh basil, finely chopped or dried
Salt and pepper to taste
Parmesan cheese, grated
Olive oil

Preheat oven to 350 degrees. Cut eggplant in half, lengthwise, then again crosswise. Make several deep slits into the meat of the eggplant without cutting through to the skin. Stuff chopped tomatoes into the slits, place garlic on top and sprinkle with basil and salt and pepper to taste. Sprinkle with Parmesan cheese. Drizzle with olive oil. Bake for 25-30 minutes.

GARLIC DRESSING
3 tbsps. apple cider vinegar
1 tbsp olive oil
1 tsp freshly squeezed lemon juice
1 clove fresh garlic, minced
1 pinch vegetable seasoning
1/2 tsp of honey

Mix all ingredients together and pour over any large mixed salad.

Soups with garlic

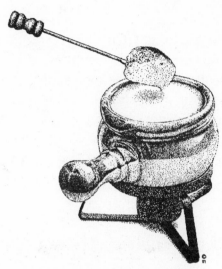

GARLIC SOUP
2 Tbs olive oil
30 large garlic cloves, chopped
2 cans chicken broth or
1 qt homemade
2 cups water
1 tsp salt
1 tsp pepper
2 bay leaves
1 fresh jalapeno pepper, seeded and chopped
1/2 cup evaporated milk
12 slices French bread
Parmesan cheese, grated

In saucepan, heat oil on medium. Add garlic and sauté until soft and golden. Add chicken broth, water, salt, pepper, bay leaves and jalapeno pepper. Simmer 5 minutes. Pour into blender and puree. Return to saucepan. Stir in the milk and heat through. Toast bread lightly. Sprinkle with Parmesan cheese and broil 3 minutes or until cheese is golden and bubbly.

AVOCADO BISQUE
2 bunches spinach, heated until just wilted but not overcooked
2 medium avocados
7 cloves fresh garlic

1/2 cup evaporated milk
1 cup chicken broth
1 tbsp. butter
1 tsp. salt
   Place everything in a blender and mix for one minute until creamy smooth. Then pour into a saucepan and cover. Heat on medium until hot, but don't boil. Serve at once. Makes a quart.

GARLIC TORTILLA SOUP

18 cloves fresh garlic
1 1/4 cups water
2 cans (11 oz. each) chicken broth
Juice of 2 limes
2 corn tortillas, cut into 1/2-inch pieces
3 egg yolks
Dash of paprika
Dash of Tabasco sauce
Pinch of cumin
Pinch of coriander
   Peel the garlic, then mix the garlic and water in a blender until well combined. Place this in a two-quart saucepan with the broth and lime juice. Simmer for half an hour. Add the tortillas and cook another ten minutes. Remove from the stove and cool until lukewarm. Slowly add the egg yolks, stirring constantly with a wire whisk. Reheat and add the paprika, cumin, coriander, and Tabasco.

TOMATO LENTIL SOUP

8 ounces dry lentils
4 cups water
1 medium onion, chopped

3 potatoes, cubed
2 to 3 carrots, sliced
1 bay leaf
1 to 2 tsps. dried sweet basil
1 tsp. dried marjoram
3 garlic cloves, finely minced
1 1/2 cups cooked chopped tomatoes
1/2 cup chopped spinach
Salt to taste

     Rinse the lentils and place in a 6-quart pot with water, onions, potatoes, carrots and the seasonings. Bring to a boil. Lower heat and let it simmer, covered for an hour or until the lentils are very soft and the vegetables are tender. Then add the tomatoes and simmer for fifteen minutes. Add the spinach and cook until just wilted. Salt to taste. A dash of lime juice adds zest. If too thick, add tomato juice or water.

OLD TESTAMENT STEW
1 cup dry lentils, rinsed
6 cups water
1 tsp. Worcestershire sauce
2 bay leaves
2 cloves garlic, minced
1/2 tsp. paprika
dash of ground cloves
1/4 tsp. black pepper
2 cups carrots, quartered
4 medium potatoes, quartered
3 medium onions, quartered
1 tbsp. cornstarch
8 oz. ground lamb meat, browned

Cover lentils with water in a large pot. Bring to a boil and cook uncovered for 30 minutes. Add the vegetables, Worcestershire sauce, bay leaves, garlic, paprika, cloves, and black pepper. Cook, covered with a lid, for another 30 minutes. Drain, reserving the broth. Set aside vegetables and lentils, then remove the bay leaves and discard. Add enough water to reserved liquid, if necessary, to equal 2 cups. Return to the pot. Whisk the cornstarch into 1/2 cup cool water until smooth, and slowly pour into the soup pot. Heat, stirring constantly until thickened. Add previously browned lamb meat, lentils, and vegetables to soup pot. Heat and serve. Serves eight.

HEARTY BEEF STEW
3 cups dry red wine
3 cups beef stock
10 garlic cloves, chopped
1 onion, chopped
3 carrots, chopped
1/4 cup olive oil
1/2 cup brandy
1/4 cup red wine vinegar
1/4 tsp. thyme
1 tbs. parsley, chopped
2 bay leaves
4 lbs. boneless beef chuck, cut into 1-inch pieces
1 cup whole garlic cloves, peeled
Cooked brown rice

Combine the wine, stock, 5 chopped garlic cloves, 1/2 of the chopped onions, carrots, 2 tbsps. of the olive oil, the brandy, vinegar and herbs in a bowl. Add the beef. Cover with plastic wrap and refrigerate overnight. Heat the remaining 2 tbsps. of oil in a large, heavy pot over medium heat. Add the remaining chopped garlic and onion and sauté until golden, for about 5 minutes. Add the beef, its marinade, and the whole garlic cloves. Cover and simmer until the beef is tender, for about two hours. Drain the cooking liquid from the beef into a large, heavy saucepan. Degrease the liquid. Boil until it's reduced to only two cups, for about an hour. Pour this sauce over the meat. Rewarm the stew over a medium heat. Simmer ten minutes. Serve over brown rice, wild rice or whole wheat noodles.

Meats with garlic

BEEF CHILI
3 cloves garlic, minced
2 large onions, finely chopped
2 tbsp olive oil
2 lbs. lean ground beef
1 8-oz can stewed tomatoes
1 4-oz can green chilies
2 cups beef stock
1 tbsp chili powder
1 tbsp ground cumin
1 tsp salt
1/2 tsp pepper
    In a large

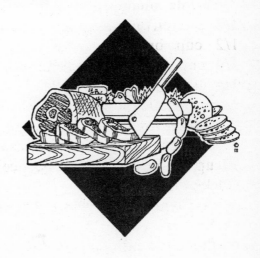

skillet, slowly brown the garlic and onions in olive oil; stir and cook until tender. Raise heat, add meat and cook until done. Add all other ingredients. Cover and reduce heat. Cook about 45 minutes more.

GRAPE LEAVES WITH LAMB
1 jar grape leaves
1 onion, chopped
2 tbsps olive oil
1 1/2 lbs ground lamb
1-2 heads garlic, peeled and chopped
Salt and pepper
4 oz pine nuts
2 cups seedless raisins
2-3 tbsps sugar
6 tsps cinnamon
4 oz. butter, melted

Preheat oven to 350 degrees. Rinse grape leaves, cut off stems and lay flat. Set aside. Sauté onion in butter or olive oil until translucent. Add lamb, crumbling as it cooks. When no longer pink, stir in garlic and season with salt and pepper to taste. Remove from heat and add pine nuts, raisins, sugar and cinnamon. Place 2-3 Tbs of the mixture in the center of each grape leaf. Fold the leaf over the filling and roll up. Place the stuffed grape leaves in a single layer in a baking dish. Dribble with melted butter. Bake for 20 minutes and serve hot. Serves 10.

DILLED SALMON
1 pound fresh salmon steaks
1 tbsp fresh dill
  Preheat oven to 425 degrees. Place the salmon steaks into a 1-quart casserole dish. Sprinkle the steaks with dill. Bake for 25 minutes, or until steaks are tender and flaky. Spoon sauce over each serving.
SAUCE
4 cloves garlic
2 egg yolks
1 tsp dry mustard
1/4 tsp white pepper
1/3 cup olive oil
2 tbsp freshly-squeezed lemon juice
  Combine garlic, egg yolks, dry mustard and white pepper in a blender, blending until smooth. With the blender running on low, slowly pour in the olive oil in a steady stream. Add fresh lemon juice. Heat in a double boiler until the mixture thickens. Serve immediately over dilled salmon.

BRAISED WHITE FISH
1 one-pound white fish
6 oz. yam
3 green onions
3 slices fresh ginger
4 cloves garlic
2 tbsps. canola oil
SAUCE
2 cups water
1 tbsp. rice wine or dry sherry

1 tbsp. hot bean paste
1 tbsp. sugar
1 tbsp. brown vinegar
1 tbsp. rice wine
1 tbsp. light soy sauce
Pinch of kelp
Clean the fish and make several diagonal slashes across each side. Peel and finely dice the yam. Chop the green onions, ginger and garlic finely. In a wok, sauté the yam in the oil for about 3 minutes until lightly colored, then place in the bottom of a casserole dish. Add the fish to the wok, sauté on both sides until lightly colored and place on top of the yam. Lightly fry the green onions, ginger and garlic in the oil and add to the casserole with the pre-mixed sauce ingredients. Bring to a rapid boil, skim any froth and residue from the surface and reduce the heat. Simmer very gently, partially covered, until the fish is tender and the stock reduced to a thick layer over the fish.

ESCARGOT IN HERBS
4 heads garlic
1/4 cup olive oil
1/4 cup butter
1 small onion, finely chopped
1 tsp fresh rosemary, finely chopped
1/4 tsp ground thyme
2 dashes nutmeg
Salt and pepper to taste
24 large canned snails
1/2 cup parsley, chopped
24 medium to large fresh mushrooms

12 pieces thin-sliced whole grain bread

     Preheat oven to 350 degrees. Peel garlic and chop into fine pieces. Place olive oil and butter in a frying pan over medium heat. When butter is melted, add onion, garlic, rosemary and thyme. Then add nutmeg, salt and pepper. Reduce heat to low and add snails and parsley; simmer for 30 minutes. While snails are simmering, clean and remove stems from mushrooms. Arrange mushroom caps upside down in a 2-inch-deep baking dish and place one snail into each mushroom cap. Pour garlic mixture over snails, cover with foil and bake for 30 minutes. Toast bread. Serve with escargots.

NEW ORLEANS CHICKEN
one 5-pound chicken
1/3 cup olive oil
1/3 cup whole wheat flour
1 1/4 cups chopped onions
1 cup chopped celery (including leaves)
1/2 cup chopped green bell pepper
3/4 cup diced garlic
10 button mushrooms
2 cups diced tomatoes
1 tbsp. finely diced jalapenos
1/2 cup tomato paste
1 tsp. crushed oregano
1 1/2 tsp. dry thyme
1 tsp. basil
1 cup dry red wine
4 cups chicken stock
Salt to taste

Cut the chicken into serving size pieces. Some of the larger pieces like the breasts may be cut into two pieces. In a two-gallon heavy saucepan heat the oil over medium high heat. Add the flour and, using a wire whisk, stir constantly until golden brown paste is achieved. When browned add the onions, celery, bell pepper, garlic, mushrooms, tomatoes, and jalapenos. Sauté 5 to 10 minutes or until the vegetables are wilted. Then add the chicken and blend well. Continue cooking an additional three minutes. Next add the tomato paste, oregano, and thyme and blend well. Add the wine and chicken stock, a little at a time, stirring constantly until all is incorporated. Bring to a low boil and reduce to simmer. Cover and cook, stirring occasionally, about one hour. Add small amounts of chicken stock should the mixture become too thick. Season to taste with salt and continue cooking until the chicken is tender. Serve over brown or wild rice. Serves six.

Garlic for Your Pet's Health

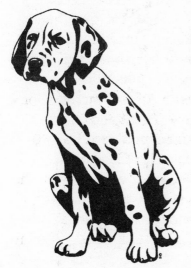

BLAND DIET FOR MILD
STOMACH DISTRESS
Cats
1 cup rice baby cereal (pre-mixed with water)
1 cup strained turkey, chicken or lamb baby food
1/2 cup low-fat cottage cheese
1/8-1/4 clove fresh-pressed garlic
    Mix ingredients and divide into 3-4 meals.

Dogs
4 cups cooked white rice
2 cups low-fat cottage cheese
2 cups boiled or broiled and diced skinless chicken
1/4 clove fresh-pressed garlic
    Mix the ingredients well and serve 3-4 times a day. This should provide enough food--more or less--for an average 20-30 pound dog for one day. Once the condition improves, wean the pet back to the regular food over a few days.

DRY SKIN SUPPLEMENT FOR DOGS
1 tbsp flax or canola oil
1 tsp brewer's yeast
1/4 clove fresh-pressed garlic
    Mix ingredients and add to food daily.

VEGETARIAN DIET FOR DOGS
3 cups boiled white rice
2 tbsps corn or safflower oil
2 large hard-boiled eggs, chopped
1/4 tsp calcium carbonate
1/4 tsp salt
1/4 tsp potassium chloride
1/2 clove fresh-pressed garlic

HYPOALLERGENIC DIET
Cats
4 oz strained lamb baby food
1 cup rice baby cereal
3/4 tsp dicalcium phosphate
1/4 clove fresh-pressed garlic

Dogs
4 oz boiled, diced lamb
2 cups boiled white rice
1 tsp safflower oil
1 1/2 tsp dicalcium phosphate
1/4 clove fresh-pressed garlic

LOW-SODIUM DIET FOR DOGS
1/4 lb lean ground beef
2 cups boiled white rice without salt
1 tbsp corn or safflower oil
2 tsp dicalcium phosphate
1/2 clove fresh-pressed garlic

Chapter 6

📖

VINEGAR FACTS & REMEDIES

from rotten apples to healing hearts

"Each patient carries his own doctor inside him. We are at our best when we give the doctor who resides within a chance to go to work." Albert Schweitzer, MD, medical missionary, 1940

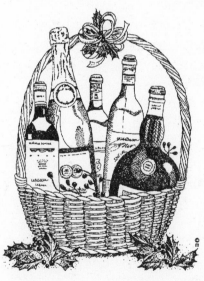

✿ PERSONAL PROFILE. HR was a retired policeman who suffered from high blood pressure. His whole life had been full of stress, and now that he had the time and money to enjoy himself, his health was shot. He was on various medications to counteract the effects of other medications. The end result was a man who was constantly tired. In true desperation, HR came to me for help. This was your basic "John Wayne" tough guy who thought green food was for babies. We talked about nutrition and options. He realized that his current life was not working and was willing to try a new program for 3 weeks. I made minimal changes to his diet, except for substituting vinegar for salt and adding considerable fresh green vegetables to his menu. HR was a notorious salt monster. He found that normal salt shakers are too stingy with salt, so he put his salt in a parmesan cheese shaker with the giant holes in the top. This guy really liked his salt!! I developed a supplement program consisting of a broad spectrum vitamin and mineral, extra vitamin C, niacin, magnesium, fish oil, and garlic. In his salt shaker, with normal size holes, he could put Lite Salt (half is potassium) or salt substitute (potassium chloride). HR acquired a taste for vinegar and became an enthusiast for the various gourmet vinegars available. He found cooking became a favorite past time and he did not miss salt one bit. He was able to stop all of his medications with his doctor's blessing because he didn't need them anymore. HR found a newly invigorating retirement life that all began with some vinegar.

Imagine a substance that is cheap and easy to make, can be taken internally for a variety of ailments, can be applied externally for all kinds of cosmetic and disinfectant purposes, and can be used in so many jobs around the house that it merits the name: "panacea". That special medicine and cleanser from Nature is apple cider vinegar, or ACV. In ACV we find the concentrated essence of the best of apples coupled with limitless by-products of bacterial fermentation, including acetic acid.

Vinegar was probably first discovered over 10,000 years ago, when our ancient ancestors found that some foods ferment into alcohol, with the next fermentation step creating vinegar. Vinegar holds a rich place in history and is mentioned often throughout the Bible. Its been said that God is always trying to make vinegar; and its the winemaker's job to interrupt the process at wine.

Vinegar was first mentioned for its medicinal value in Babylonia around 7000 years ago.

Hippocrates, the father of modern medicine, prescribed vinegar often for his patients 2400 years ago. Since the days of the Old Testament, laborers would add vinegar and salt to water to create their own "Gatorade" drink to keep their energy levels up while sweating under the hot sun. Ancient Persian physicians would recommend a drink of vinegar, lime juice, and sour fruit juice to help prevent fatty accumulation in the body. Early Greek, Roman, and Asian physicians would use vinegar to treat scurvy, digestive problems, and bile reduction. In 1958, Dr. D.C. Jarvis resurrected American interest in vinegar through his popular book FOLK MEDICINE.

Vinegar has played a major role in human history. The Roman army that once conquered much of the known world, relied heavily on vinegar to survive the changes in climate and combat stress. Roman soldiers also used fire and vinegar alternately to heat and contract rocks in order to break their way through the Alps mountains. Cleopatra, Queen of Egypt, won a major bet by dissolving a pearl in a glass of vinegar and drinking it, thus proving that she could consume a meal worth a fortune. Louis the XIII of France was charged 1.3 million francs for the vinegar used to cool his armies' cannons during battle.

Lacking refrigeration, our ancestors either had to eat the entire animal in one sitting or figure out some way to preserve the meat lest it rot. Vinegar solutions, or "pickling", along with salting and smoking became the favorite ways to keep foods from rotting.

During the Black Plague of the Middle Ages, people were spared from the plague by breathing through a cloth soaked in vinegar, thanks to its antiseptic properties. Once the industrial era began gearing up in the 18th century, cities throughout Europe became very large and smelly, since indoor plumbing was a rare commodity. To tolerate the stench of raw sewage on the streets, genteel people would walk or ride through London and Paris with sponges soaked in vinegar held to their nose, taking advantage of the pungent but pleasant aroma from vinegar. These sponges were carried in small silver boxes, or vinaigrettes, or in special compartments in the heads of walking canes.

The term "vinegar" is derived from French words "vinaigre" meaning "sour wine". Yet looking further back into Old French, we find that "aigre" could also have meant "eager, sharp, or biting". Thus, its name may not be some derogatory "sour wine" as much as a compliment "sharp wine".

HOW IS IT MADE?

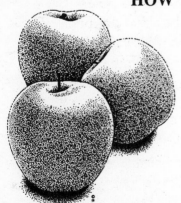

Vinegar is obtained from the fermentation of alcohol. Basically, when carbohydrate foods are "eaten" by tiny organisms (yeasts of the genus Saccharomyces), the first action is to convert sugars into alcohol. If allowed to continue to ferment, the next stage involves a different set of bacteria, called acetobacter, which "eat" the alcohol and give off the by-product of acetic acid, along with thousands of other "congeners" or unidentified by-products. Now we have vinegar, which has been made around the world in nearly every culture for longer than the Pyramids have been standing.

FOOD PRODUCT	ALCOHOL BY-PRODUCT	VINEGAR
grapes	wine	wine vinegar
apples	hard cider	cider vinegar
corn, rye	malt liquor	malt vinegar
rice	sake	rice vinegar

Vinegar usually has an acid content of between 4 and 8 percent, which means that there is somewhere between 4 to 8 grams of acetic acid per 100 cubic centimeters (cc) of vinegar.
Unfortunately, the vast majority of vinegar sold in the U.S. is distilled. In this last, and highly unnecessary, phase, the processor exposes the vinegar to heat and then catches the vapors. The result is a light amber colored apple cider vinegar that looks more like beer and is a mere "cadaver" of the nutrient-dense ACV before the distillation process.

The consumer is as much to blame for this distillation phase as the manufacturer. We buy food with our eyes. The unprocessed ACV is dark, cloudy, and has spider web things (Mother of Vinegar bacteria colonies) floating through it. It doesn't look as appealing to the untrained eye as

the translucent distilled ACV. For the remainder of
this chapter, all benefits of ACV are for the
unprocessed variety. You may have to go to your
nearest health food store to get this kind of vinegar.
There are some mail order companies listed in the
appendix who sell unprocessed vinegar. When
using vinegar for cleaning purposes, the cheaper
distilled versions of ACV are perfect.

Several varieties of vinegar are
manufactured. Wine vinegars, produced in grape-
growing regions, are used for salad dressings and
relishes. Tarragon and raspberry vinegars are
flavored by the addition of the herb or fruit. Malt
vinegar, popular in Great Britain, is known for its
earthy quality. White vinegar is made from
industrial alcohol. Because of its less distinctive
flavor, it is often used as a preservative. Piquant
rice vinegar is used in Oriental countries. Aged,
richly-flavored balsamic vinegar is an Italian
specialty.

In industry, vinegar can be made from wood
alcohol, which produces a potent solvent. This
industrial vinegar can be combined with alcohol to
form acetates, which are used throughout industry
as solvents. Industrial vinegar is combined with
cellulose (fiber) to form cellulose acetate, which is
the starting process to make rayon and other
artificial fibers and for photographic film.

ACV may be used as an ingredient of sweet-
and-sour sauces for meat and vegetable dishes, as a
minor ingredient in candies, or as an ingredient in
baking for the leavening process. Vinegar is also
added to milk, if sour milk is needed in a home

recipe. Commercially and in the home, the most common use of vinegar is in the making of salad dressings. About 98% of American homes have vinegar in the kitchen. Sales have increased by about 10% in the last decade, possibly because Americans are seeking "simple solutions for complex problems". Vinegar is to panaceas what Abraham Lincoln was to public speakers--one of the best.

WHAT'S IN VINEGAR?

For 99% of the 7000 years that vinegar has been used medicinally, no one knew why it relieved health problems. In recent years, various proponents of vinegar have offered their own explanation of why vinegar seems to prevent and reverse so many common diseases. On the surface, ACV seems to be a rather unimpressive food.

> **8 ounces of ACV contains:**
> 98.8% water
> 34 calories
> no fat
> trace of protein
> trace of pectin fiber
> 14.2 grams of carbohydrate
> 14 mg calcium (less than 2% of the USRDA)
> 22 mg phosphorus
> 1.4 mg iron
> 2 mg sodium
> 240 mg potassium (half of what is in a banana)

When we talk about commercially distilled vinegar, these numbers all go down to near zero, with potassium cut to 36 mg, which is an 85% loss in potassium. In my opinion, the real reasons that ACV is so full of health giving properties is:

1) pH, its acid content

2) active bacteria

3) bacterial by-products, also known as congeners, which literally means "from the same source or stock".

1) pH. One of the reasons that vinegar is so healthy is that it helps to rectify the unhealthy acidic environment found inside most Americans, from our poor diet, stress, and sedentary lifestyle. Acids and bases are categories of chemicals based upon their "potential hydrogens", or pH. Acids were recognized originally by their sour taste in water and because they could attack and dissolve some metals. The word acid is derived from acetum

(Latin, "vinegar"). Bases were substances that were usually soapy to the touch and that could react with acids in water to form neutral salts.

Baking soda, or sodium bicarbonate, is a common base or alkaline agent in your kitchen. Vinegar or lemon juice is a common acid used in the kitchen. Neutral substances, or salts and water, are given the pH number of 7. The pH of acids ranges from 1 to 7 (1 is the strongest) and bases from 7 to 14 (14 is the strongest). Vinegar is a strongly acidic solution with a pH of around 2, which is why Cleopatra was able to dissolve a pearl in a glass of vinegar. By the way, I haven't tried this experiment.

The very important but confusing aspect of eating an acidic food, like vinegar or lemon juice, is that it creates an alkaline environment in the body. What happens is the acid gets to the small intestines, where the pancreas detects acid in the gut, then releases a bicarbonate buffer into the bloodstream. The bloodstream of a healthy adult has a pH which is mildly alkaline, about 7.41. There are many medical textbooks which spend a great deal of time teaching doctors how to finely balance pH in the human body. Deviations from the normal can create disease or death. Even slight changes in pH in the body may lead to degenerative diseases, such as cancer and mental illness. Balancing pH in the body is essential, though it may not be sufficient to cure a disease.

pH in the body is dictated by: diet, breathing, water intake, stress, exercise.

A diet rich in fruits, vegetables, whole grains, and legumes will help bring the body into a healthy pH of about 7.41. A typical American diet of meat, ice cream, and sugar will bring the pH lower, into an acidic range, which creates all kinds of health problems. Shallow breathing brings about an acidic body, while deep breathing and exercise help to bring the body into the alkaline range. Drinking lots of clean water also helps to reverse the body's natural tendency to become more acidid, through lactic acid production from energy metabolism. Stress also creates the more unhealthy acidic environment in the blood.

Also, as we mature, the body loses its ability to make enough hydrochloric acid in the stomach. Regular use of ACV helps to insure a strong acid environment in the stomach, which improves the digestion and absorption of foods as well as protecting us against viruses and bacteria that enter the body through the gut.

2) Bacteria. When Louis Pasteur noticed that heat killed off the tiny organisms under his microscope, he began a fervent quest to kill off all bacteria. Experts of those days reasoned "if bacteria causes disease, then let's get rid of all bacteria." On his death bed, after a brilliant and productive career, Pasteur conceded "it is the terrain". In other words, the terrain, or the human host, is more important than the bacteria itself. Actually, as our microscopes have become more powerful, we find trillions of bacteria everywhere-- and some of them are very helpful for your health.

Bacteria and yeast are tiny organisms that you cannot see with the naked eye. You could easily put a thousand bacteria on the period at the end of this sentence. The objective of any bacteria is simple: survive long enough to reproduce. Some bacteria are parasitic, such as staphylococcus and salmonella that create havoc in food poisoning. Other bacteria are symbiotic, meaning they contribute something to the relationship of living within another organism, kind of like "paying rent". A cow cannot digest the hay that it eats, but the bacteria in the cow's stomach can digest the hay. The bacteria gets a place to live and a conveyor belt constantly bringing in a food supply, while the cow gets nourishment from a food that is otherwise indigestible.

There are about 50 billion bacteria in a pound of human fecal matter. Some of the bacteria in your gut help to make vitamins, like K and biotin. Some of the bacteria help to build a protective gut lining to prevent infections. Some bacteria, as from yogurt, give off by-products like blastolysin, that bolster the body's immune system. In other words, bacteria are not all bad. Some of them are downright helpful, such as the bacteria in ACV.

Lactobacillus acidophilus is the bacteria strain added to milk to create the fermented end product of yogurt. Yogurt has been scientifically proven to have many health values beyond milk, simply because of the bacteria and their by-products. Vinegar is to apples what yogurt is to milk. There are other examples of fermented foods eaten around the world. Another reason that ACV is so healthy is the bacteria it contributes to encourage a healthy gut.

FOOD PRODUCT	FERMENTED END PRODUCT
milk	yogurt
milk	kefir
wheat	sourdough bread
cabbage	sauerkraut
soybeans	tempeh
apples	apple cider vinegar

"Mother-of-vinegar" is the mass of sticky scum which forms on top of cider when alcohol turns into vinegar. As the fermentation progresses, "mother" forms a gummy, stringy, floating lump. "Mother" is formed by the beneficial bacteria which creates vinegar. These bacteria are a major reason why vinegar is so good for your health. These bacteria are not found in regular commerical distilled vinegar.

3) Bacteria by-products. When the old time "moonshiners" would brew up a batch of liquor, they oftentimes blew up the distillation unit because the yeast would be fermenting the corn mash too fast. When yeast or bacteria ferment a food, they create alcohol, gases, and thousands of different "congeners" as by-products of metabolism. These congeners not only provide the characteristic flavor found in many beers, wines, and liquors; they also influence the relative severity of the hangover.

We now know that when bacteria ferment food in our gut, the by-products can be anything from the essential vitamin biotin to a nasty substance that may create arthritis. ACV seems to contain not only thousands of substances that are found in apples, but also thousands of other unidentified substances formed in the fermentation process. The below list helps you to appreciate how complex whole foods really are. Another reason that ACV prevents and reverses many ailments is this lengthy list of "minor dietary constituents", some of which are probably very therapeutic and the possible by-products from bacterial fermentation.

WHAT'S IN A FRESH WHOLE CLEAN APPLE?

[from "Handbook of Phytochemical Constituents of Generally Regarded as Safe (GRAS) Herbs"]

abscisic-acid fr nap
cis-2, trans-4-abscisic-acid bk nap
trans-abscisic-acid fr nap
acetic-acid
acetic-acid-amyl-ester
acetaldehyde
acetone
n-alpha-acetyl-agginine sh nap
adenine rt nap
alpha-alanine fr
beta-alanine fr
alanine 70-435 fr usa
aluminum 0.4-129 fr aas usg
alpha-aminobutyric-acid
ammonia (NH3) 235-1,029 EP(FR)
amygdalin 6,000-13,800 sd
amyl-acetate
amyl-butyrate
amyl-propionate
aniline 1.7 ep(fr) nap
aniline 1.5 fr nap
arabinose
arginine 60-373 fr usa
arsenic 0.00055-0.43 fr aas usg
ascorbic-acid 20-402 fr usa
ascorbidase
ash 2,300-43,000 fr aas usg
asparagine 171 fr
aspartic-acid 210-2,115 fr usa
avicularin fr nap

barium 0.22-8.6 fr usg
benzoic-acid
3,4-benzopyrene fr nap
benzyl-acetate
benzyl-amine 0.6 ep(fr) nap
benzylamine 0.3-3.0 fr nap
biotin
boron 1-110 fr aas bob usg
bromine <1 fr aas
butanol
n-butanol
1-butanol
2-butanol
butyl-acetate
butyl-butyrate
butyl-caproate
butyl-propionate
butyl-valerianate
i-butyl-octanoate
i-butyl-propioante
n-butyl-decanoate
n-butyl-formate
n-butyl-n-hexanoate
n-butyl-octanoate
n-butyl-propionate
cadmium <0.002-0.0258 fr aas usg
caffeetannin
caffeic-acid 85-1,270 fr crc(fsn)
calcium 43-750 (-1,376) fr aas usg
calcium-oxalate
caproaldehyde
caproic-acid-amyl-ester
caprylic-ester
carobohydrate 152,250-948,550 fr
beta-carotene 0-76 fr
carotenoids 0-126 fr
catalase
d-catechin fr nap
chlorogenic-acid fr nap
chlorophyll 0-1 fr
chromium 0.005-0.3 fr aas usg
citric-acid
citramalic-acid
cobalt <0.005-0.043 fr aas usg
copper 0.24-4 fr aas usg
coumaric-acid

p-coumaric-acid 15-460 fr crc(fsn)
n-coumaryl-quinic-acid
p-coumaryl-quinic-acid fr nap
creatine sh nap
cutin ep(fr) nap
cyanidin lf nap
cyanidin-3-arabinoside
cyanidin-7-arabinoside
cynanidin-3,5-diglucoside
cy nap
cyanidin-3-galactoside
cystine 30-187
i-decanoic-acid
n-decanol
decenoic-acid
i-decyl-acetate
dehydroascorbic-acid
diastase
diethylamine 3 fr nap
digalactosyl-diglyceride 49-107 fr
3-beta-19-alpha-dihydroxy-2-oxo-urs-12-en-28-oic-acid 1,000 wd nap
dihydroxytricarballylic-acid 1 fr
diphosphatidyl-glycerol 4-6 fr
eo 25-35 fr
l-epicatechin fr nap
5,6-epoxy-10'-apo-5,6-dihydro-beta-carotene-3,10'-diol 20,000 ep(fr) nap
estragole tr eo
estrone 0.10-0.13 sd nap
ethanol
ethyl-acetate
ethylamine 3 fr nap
ethyl-butyrate
ethyl-caproate
ethyl-crotonate
ethyl-decenoate
ethyl-dodecanoate
ethyl-hexanoate
ethyl-isobutyrate
ethyl-methylbutyrate
ethyl-nonanoate
ethyl-octanoate
ethyl-pentanoate
ethyl-phenacetate
ethyl-propionate
ethyl-valerianate

farnesene ep(fr) nap
fat 3,210-34,200 fr fnf
ped
fat 180,00-230,000 sd
ferulic-acid 4-95 fr
crc(fsn)
fiber 131,000 fr ped
fiber 5,200-49,636 fr usa
fluorine <0.1-2.1 fr aas
folacin 0.02-0.2 fr usa
formic-acid
fructose 50,100-60,800 fr
fumaric-acid
galactanase
galactaric-acid
d-galacturonic-acid 13-54
geraniol
d-glucitol
glucocerebroside 34-49
d-gluconic-acid
glucose 17,200-18,200 fr
glutamic-acid 156-1,244
fr
glutamine 20
glyceric-acid
glycine 80-497
glycolic-acid
glyoxylic-acid
guanidine sh nap
guanidinoacetic-acid sh
nap
gamma-
guanidinobutramide sh
nap
gamma-guanidinobutyric-
acid sh nap
gamma-
guanidinopropionic-acid
sh nap
guanidinosuccinic-acid sh
nap
hemicellulose
heptacosane
n-heptanoic-acid
heptenoic-acid
2-heptanol
n-heptanol
n-hex-1-en-3-ol
cis-n-hex-3-en-1-ol
trans-n-hex-2-en-1-ol
trans-n-hex-3-en-1-ol
hexacosanol
n-hexanol
7-hexanoic-acid
i-hexanoic-acid
hexanol

2-hexenal
trans-2-hexenoic-acid
hexyl-acetate
hexyl-butyrate
hexyl-formate
n-hehyl-n-hexanoate
n-hexyl-octanoate
n-hexyl-propionate
histidine 30-187 fr
p-hydroxybenzoic-acid fr
nap
hydroxycinnamic-acid
1,340 fr
4-hydroxymethylproline
3-hydroxy-octyl-beta-d-
glucoside fr nap
19-hydroxyursolic-acid pl
jsg
20-hydroxyursolic-acid pl
jsg
19-hydroxyursonic-acid pl
jsg
hyperin
hyperoside fr nap
idaein
indole-3-acetic-acid pl pas
inositol
iodine
iron 1.1-123 fr aas usa usg
isoamyl-butyrate
isoamyl-propionate
isobutyl-acetate
isobutyl-butyrate
isobutyl-formate
isochlorogenic-acid pl pas
isocitric-acid
isoleucine 50-497 fr
isopropyl-butyrate
isoquercitrin fr nap
jasmonic-acid fr nap
kilocalories 3,419 fr ped
lactic-acid
lauric-acid 10-63 fr
lead 0.002-64 fr aas usg
lecithin
leucine 120-746 fr
linolenic-acid 870-5,411
fr omega-3
alpha-linolenic-acid 180-
1,120 fr omega-3
lithium 0.044-0.172 fr
usg
lutein 0.4-5 fr jaf37:657
luteoxanthin fr nap
lysine 20-746 fr

magnesium 48-478 (-
860) fr aas usa usg
l-malic-acid
malvidin-monoglycoside
manganese 0-29 fr aas usg
mannose
mercury 0.00011-0.02 fr
aas usg
methanol
methionine 20-124
methyl-acetate
methyl-2-xi-acetoxy-20-
beta-hydroxy-ursonate
ep(fr)
methylamine 4.5 ep(fr)
nap
2-methyl-but-2-en-1-al fr
nap
2-methyl-but-3-en-1-ol fr
nap
d-2-methylbutan-1-ol
2-methylbutan-2-ol
methyl-butyrate
methyl-caproate
2-methyl-2,3-epoxy-
pentane fr nap
24-methylene-cholesterol
po nap
methyl-formate
methyl-guanidine sh nap
6-methyl-hepten-5-en-2-
one fr nap
methyl-hexanoate
n-methyl-beta-
phenethylamine 1.2 fr
nap
methyl-propionate
methyl-2-methyl-butyrate
methyl-i-pentanoate
methyl-n-pentanoate
2-methylpentan-2-ol
n-methyl-phenethylamine
1.3 ex(fr) nap
n-methyl-phenethylamine
1.2 fr nap
gamma-methyl-proline
2-methyl-propen-1-al fr
nap
methyl-vinyl-ketone fr nap
mevalonic-acid 30-36 fr
molybdenum 0.077-0.43
fr usg
monogalactosyl-diglyceride
12-42
1-mono-linolein sd nap
mufa 150-935 fr usa

myoinositol 4,500 po nap
myristic-acid 20-124 fr
neochlorogenic-acid
neoxanthin ep(fr) nap
niacin 1-7 fr
nickel 0.004-0.645 fr aas
usg
nitrogen 280-4,000 fr aas
nonacosane
d-l-nonacosanol
n-nonanoic-acid
n-nonanol-2-nonanol
nonenoic-acid
1-nonyl-acetate
octacosanol
octa-cis-3-cis-5-dien-1-ol
eo nap
octa-trans-3-cis-5-dien-1-
ol eo nap
octa-cis-3-cis-5-dien-1-ol-
acetate eo nap
octa-trans-3-cis-5-dien-1-
ol-acetate eo nap
n-octanone
n-octanol-2-octanol
octenoic-acid
1-octyl-acetate
oleic-acid 140-871 fr
oxalic-acid
oxaloacetic-acid
alpha-oxoglutaric-acid
palmitic-acid 480-2,986
fr
palmitoleic-acid 10-62 fr
pantothenic-acid 1-4 fr
usa
pectase
pectin 1,400-66,585 fr
usa
pectin-demethoxyxylase
n-pentanoic-acid
i-pentanoic-acid
pentanol
i-pentanol
2-pentanol
3-pentanol
n-pentenoic-acid
n-pentyl-amine 0.3 fr nap
pentyl-butyrate
n-pentyl-decanoate
n-pentyl-formate
i-pentyl-formate
pentyl-hexanoate
n-pentyl-2-
methylbutyrate
i-pentyl-i-pentanoate

n-pentyl-octanoate
peroxidase
2-phenethylacetate
phenolics 1,100-3,400
phenylalanine 50-311 fr
phloretamide fr nap
phloretin 1f jad
phloretin-4'-o-beta-d-
glucopyranoside 6,486 fr
nap
phloretin-xyloglucoside fr
nap
phlorizin
phosphatidylic-acid 3-6 fr
phosphatidyl-choline 189-
214 fr
phosphatidyl-
ethanolamine 101-124 fr
phosphatidyl-glycerol 8-
27 fr
phosphatidyl-inositol 53-
59 fr
phosphatidyl-serine 4 fr
phosphorus 68-925 (-
1,548) fr aas ped usg
phytosterols 120-745 fr
usa
pipecolinic-acid
polygalactosyl-diglyceride
polygalacturonase
polyphenolase
pomolic-acid pl jsg
pomonic-acid pl jsg
potassium 1,110-12,140
(-17,630) fr aas usg
procyanidins 1f nap
proline 20-435
propanol
2-propanol
n-propanol
i-propanol
n-propionic-acid
propyl-acetate
propyl-butyrate
propyl-formate
propyl-2-methylbutyrate
propyl-n-pentanoate
propyl-propionate
protein 1,870-12,800 fr
ped
protocatechuic-acid fr nap
pufa 1,050-6,535 fr usa
pyrrolidine 1.5 ep(fr) nap
pyroxidine
pyruvic-acid
quercetin 58-263 pc pam

quercetin-arabinoside
quercetin-3-o-alpha-
arabinofuranoside pl jsg
quercetin-3-o-alpha-
galactoside ep(fr) nap
quercetin-3-o-beta-d-
glucoside pl jsg
quercetin-3-
rhamnoglucoside
quercetin-3-o-rhamnoside
pl jsg
quercetin-3-rutinoside
quercetin-3-o-xyloside
ep(fr) nap
quercitrin fr nap
l-quinic-acid
reynoutrin fr nap
riboflavin 1 fr
rubidium 0.27-10 fr aas
rutin tr ep(fr) nap
selenium 0.000055-
0.00043 fr usg
serline 80-497 fr usa
sfa 580-3,610 fr usa
shikimic-acid
silicon 1-70 fr aas
silver 0.011-0.086 fr usg
sinapic-acid fr nap
sodium 0-133 fr usg
sorbitol 1f nap
stearic-acid 70-435 fr
strontium 0.165-8.6 fr usg
succinic-acid
sucrose 24,000-36,200 fr
sugar 60,100-166,000 fr
sulfur 1.65-23 fr usg
tetradecenyl-acetate 1f
nap
tetradecyl-acetate 1f nap
thiamin 1-2 fr ped
threonine 30-435 fr
titanium 0.055-3 fr usg
alpha-tocopherol 2-37 fr
tot usa
triacontanol
triglyceride 45-50
1,3,3,-trimethyl-dioxa-
2,7-bicyclo(2,2,1)heptane
fr nap
tryptophan 20-124 fr
tyrosine 40-249 fr
uronic-acid 7-1,440 fr
ursolic-acid ep(fr) nap
valine 40-560 fr
vit-b6 1-3 fr

vomifoliol-1-o-beta-d-
xylopyranosyl-6-o-beta-d-
glucopyranoside fr nap
water   809,000-896,000
fr usg
xylose
zinc 0-35 fr aas usg
zirconium 0.22-0.86 fr
usg
Many entries derived from
Hulme, aas=acta agric
scand suppl, 22:1980
water=86%

In summary, ACV is an amazing gift from Nature--a phenomenally versatile substance that should be in every home, kitchen, first aid kit, workshop, and pharmacy. Enjoy the following remedies from this wonderous food!!

AMAZING MEDICAL FACTS ABOUT VINEGAR

The difference between modern medicine and folk medicine is that we can scientifically document **how** modern medicine works, but we don't yet know how folk remedies work. ACV has the "pole position" in folk medicine. Thousands of years of successful use in millions of people can't be all wrong.

However, since no drug company is going to spend the time and money to research a product, like vinegar, which cannot be patented, there is precious little interest among scientists to study the effects of vinegar in humans. Yet, in spite of the lack of funding and respect for vinegar, there have been a few studies, and here are the best of the best.

Stings and bites. Stings from jellyfish and other creatures are no trivial matter. They can easily send a person to the hospital. Numerous medical journals now endorse the use of vinegar as the best first aid for fresh stings. Australians are very familiar with jellyfish stings, which can cause pain, nausea, headache, chills and possibly even heart attack and death. Medical researchers find that splashing vinegar on the sting immediately afterward will substantially reduce swelling and other symptoms.[1] Stings of bees, wasps, jellyfish, and many other bothersome creatures can be eased by soaking the hurting area in full-strength vinegar. For best results, the vinegar should be applied immediately after the encounter.

Blood glucose regulation. One of the more important aspects of overall health is maintaining the proper level of sugar in the blood. Too much sugar in the blood and diabetes sets in, with gangrene, kidney failure, heart disease, and other problems to contend with. If blood sugar is slightly elevated, the person throws off prostaglandin balance, which is one of the most potent substances made in the body. Too little sugar in the blood and the person will experience headache, jitters, loss of memory, anxiety, irritability, and weakness. Healthy blood glucose runs around 80 to 100 mg per 100 ml of blood. The vast majority of Americans ride a lifetime rollercoaster of too high and too low blood sugar and thus are constantly playing "Russian roulette" by eating too much sugar, not enough fiber, not enough chromium and other nutrients for sugar regulation. But scientists find that a simple salad dressing which includes vinegar can help to stabilize blood sugar levels during and after a meal.[2]

Are you absorbing your vitamins? Americans purchase nearly $6 billion each year of vitamin supplements and health food. This industry is growing, which is a positive sign that Americans are beginning to take charge of their health. Unfortunately, not all vitamin pills are created alike or even useful. Some vitamins, minerals, herbs, and other pills are manufactured under intense pressure, then coated with shellac or wax to ensure a longer shelf life. These vitamins essentially become like a rock, which passes through the intestinal tract undigested and therefore wasted. However, you can accurately determine how well absorbed your vitamins will be by dropping your pills in a glass of lukewarm dilute vinegar water. Scientists find that this test nicely predicts how well you are absorbing that pill.[3]

Food borne infections reduced. While Americans occasionally experience a bout of food poisoning, other countries around the world are under constant siege with life-threatening bacteria and other parasites in the food and water supply. Ethiopian researchers found that vinegar was the champion at killing a tough cyst (Cysticercus bovis), which is the nearly-invincible egg phase for some intestinal parasites. The only thing more lethal to these parasites than vinegar was intense close X-rays!![4] If you are going out to dinner or, especially if you are visiting a foreign country, make sure that you have a 1-2 teaspoon "cocktail" of vinegar before dining on any questionable food.

SECRET FAMILY RECIPE FOR HEALTH

My favorite health-promoting salad dressing can be made from 1/4 cup vinegar, 1/4 cup flax oil, and 1/8 cup honey. Mix well and serve at the evening meal to keep the whole family in good health. For added flavoring, use spices: Lite Salt (half potassium), garlic powder, onion powder, mustard, basil, and thyme. Darn near cures whatever ails you.

REMEDIES FOR HEALTH & HOME

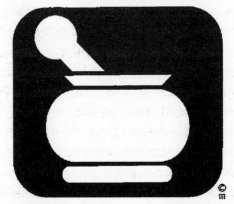

The acid content of vinegar makes it useful for a wide range of cleaning chores and other tasks around the home. Inexpensive, with no dangerous fumes or additives, a gallon of cheap commercial distilled white or apple cider vinegar can replace a number of other containers found around the house. Cleaners that you make yourself are cheaper, safe, natural, and easy on the environment.

As with all cleaning products, test these vinegar solutions on cleaning problems before using them. Always try them out on an inconspicuous area of rugs, upholstery, or clothing. Vinegar can dissolve pre-existing wax on furniture and floors. Use very small amounts to clean and shine, stronger solutions to remove wax buildup and heavy dirt.

Many folk recipes combine vinegar with other household supplies. Commercial chemical cleaners are not always as environmentally safe as more natural, organic compounds. A number of popular substances have been used in combination with vinegar to make spectacular cleaners. To vinegar, add:

Baking soda to absorb odors, deodorize, and as a mild abrasive.

Borax to disinfect, deodorize, and stop the growth of mold.

Chalk for a mild, non abrasive cleaner.

Oil to preserve and shine.

Pumice to remove stains or polish surfaces.

Salt for a mild abrasive.

Washing soda to cut heavy grease.

Wax to protect and shine.

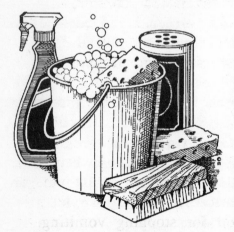

CAUTION: When some ingredients are added to a vinegar solution, a frothy foam is produced. This is a natural chemical reaction, and is not dangerous in an open container. DO NOT SEAL A FOAMING VINEGAR MIXTURE IN A TIGHTLY CAPPED CONTAINER!

FROM A TO Z, EVERYTHING YOU CAN DO WITH VINEGAR

Acne. Make a mixture of 2 teaspoons of plain or herbal apple cider vinegar in 1 cup of water and dab on blemishes several times a day after washing. Old herbals recommend a mixture of onion and vinegar for blemishes.

Age spots, also called liver spots, may fade if you wipe them daily with onion juice and vinegar. 1 teaspoon onion juice and 2 teaspoons vinegar would be mixed together and applied with a soft cloth. Or, 1/2 a fresh onion can be dipped into a dish of vinegar and then rubbed across the skin. It takes a few weeks for the spot to begin to fade.

Air freshener. Put the following into a pump spray bottle: 1 teaspoon baking soda, 1 tablespoon vinegar, and 2 cups of water. After the foaming stops, put on the lid and shake well. Spray this mixture into the air for instant freshness.

Aluminum utensils cleaned. Remove dark stains from the inside of aluminum utensils by adding vinegar to boiling water and simmering until clean.

Animal acceptance. Dairy farmers reports that a new cow is quickly accepted into the herd when she is sprayed with a solution of vinegar and water. Actually, if you spill vinegar anywhere near livestock, they will eat the soil to get at the vinegar.

Anti-emetic (vomit stopper). Clove vinegar is especially good for stopping vomiting. Its use dates back to China more than 2,000 years ago where it was also considered an aphrodisiac.

Antiseptic action. Antiseptics are chemicals applied to body surfaces to reduce the infectious growth of bacteria, viruses, and fungi. Vinegar has been one of history's favorite antiseptics, recommended by Hippocrates to Pasteur.

Ants repelled. Ants will stay away from a kitchen or any area wiped down or sprayed with a solution of equal parts water and vinegar.

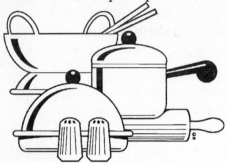

Appliances sparkle if cleaned with a vinegar and borax combination. Mix 1 teaspoon borax, 1/4 cup vinegar, and 2 cups hot water and put it into a spray bottle. Spray it on greasy smears and wipe off with a cloth or sponge.

Arthritis. D.C. Jarvis, M.D., reports that drinking 2 1/2 teaspoons of apple cider vinegar in a glass of water at each meal helps to alleviate arthritis.

Asthma can be relieved by combining the advantages of acupressure with the benefits of apple cider vinegar. Use a wide rubber band to hold gauze pads, which have been soaked in vinegar, to the inside of the wrists.

Athlete's foot itching relieved. Soak socks or hose in vinegar water. Mix 1 part vinegar with 5 parts water and soak for 30 minutes before washing as usual.

Athlete's Foot. Relieve the itching of athlete's foot by rinsing the feet several times a day with plain or herbal apple cider vinegar.

Baths. Adding either plain or herbal vinegar to bath water does for the entire body what vinegar skin tonics do for the face. Your skin responds favorably to having the proper acid, or pH balance.

Vinegar in the bath water relaxes, soothes, cleanses, and removes itching, flaking skin. Use plain apple cider, rice, or wine vinegar or an herbal vinegar, adding 1/4 to 1 cup vinegar to the bath water. Herbal vinegars also make delightful after-bath body splashes for softening the skin; use full-strength or diluted.

Birth control. Attempts at family planning have been going on for thousands of years. Some ancient methods, though crude, were based on sound ideas. For example, women were advised to put honey, olive oil, or oil of cedar in their vaginas. The stickiness of these substances might slow the movement of sperm into the uterus. Wads of soft wool soaked in lemon juice or vinegar were used as tampons, making the vagina sufficiently acidic to kill the sperm.

Brass and copper are cleaned with 2 teaspoons salt, 1 tablespoon flour, and enough vinegar to make a paste. First, mix the salt and flour together. Next, add vinegar until a thick paste is formed. Then use the paste to scrub the metal, rinse, and buff dry. Add some extra salt for hard jobs, or some extra flour for a softer paste.

Brass and copper cleaner. Combining equal parts of lemon juice and vinegar. Wipe it on with a paper towel, then polish with a soft, dry cloth.

Brass and copper will sparkle and tarnish will melt away if wiped down with 2 tablespoons catsup and 1 tablespoon vinegar. Polish until completely dry with a clean cloth.

Brighten carpet. Rejuvenate carpet colors by brushing with a mixture of 1 cup vinegar in 1 gallon of water.

Brushes hardened with old, dried-in paint may be softened by boiling them in vinegar. Simply cover them with boiling vinegar and let them stand for 1 hour. Then heat the vinegar and brushes until the vinegar comes to a gentle boil. Simmer for 20 minutes. Rinse well, working the softened paint out of the bristles. For extremely heavy paint residue, you may need to repeat the process.

Burns and Sunburn. To alleviate the pain of minor burns and sunburn, including lye burns, pat cold apple cider vinegar on affected area every 20 minutes.

Calming effect. Lavender makes a vinegar that is pleasantly aromatic and useful for fighting off anxiety attacks. The haunting scent of lavender has long been associated with headache relief and calming of stressed nerves.

Car chrome shines up fast if polished with vinegar.

Carpet stains lifted. Dissolve 2 tablespoons salt and 2 tablespoons borax in 1/2 cup vinegar. Rub this into carpet stains and let it dry. Vacuum up the residue.

Carpet stains removed. While stain is still fresh, apply a mixture of 1 part vinegar to 3 parts water and let it stand for a few minutes. Sponge from the center out and blot with a dry cloth.

Cats kept out of the garden. Soak pieces of paper in vinegar and put around the garden.

Cement removed from hands. To clean up hands after working in cement or concrete, wash hands in vinegar, then rinse with water.

Chapped Skin. Chapped hands heal quickly when treated with a homemade mixture of equal parts rich hand cream and vinegar. Use it every time you wash your hands.

Check calcium supplements. To check the absorbability of calcium supplements, drop them into vinegar. If they dissolve quickly, then they are of good quality.

Chewing gum dissolved and decals removed by saturating them with vinegar. Vinegar removes gum from fabric, carpet, and upholstery. If the vinegar is heated, it will work faster.

Clean bottles, jars, and vases. Remove chalky mineral film on bottles, jars, and vases by pouring in vinegar, letting it stand for several minutes. Then shake or brush vigorously. To use in a dishwasher, place a cup of vinegar on the bottom rack, run the machine for 3 to 5 minutes, replace the vinegar with a fresh cup, then complete the dishwashing cycle with dishwasher detergent.

Clothes get whiter. Add 1 1/2 cups vinegar to rinse water to brighten laundry.

Coffee and tea stains cleaned from glass and china. Boil vinegar in glass coffee pots once a week, wash, and rinse. Equal parts vinegar and salt removes stains from cups.

Colds are banished. Soak an eight-inch square of brown paper cut from a paper grocery bag in apple cider vinegar. When the paper is saturated sprinkle it with pepper and bind to the chest with cloth strips, pepper side of the paper next to the skin. After 20 minutes, remove the paper and wash the chest, being careful not to become chilled.

Congestion relief. Eucalyptus is the source of the eucalyptol which makes some cough drops so effective. Steam from vinegar which has absorbed the aromatic oil of this herb helps to clear a stuffy head or a clogged respiratory system. A popular over-the-counter salve for relieving the stiffness and swelling of arthritis and rheumatism carries the distinctive aroma of eucalyptus.

Cooking odors eliminated. Prevent the odor of boiling cabbage by adding a little vinegar to the cooking water. To remove the odor of fish or onions from your hands, wipe them with vinegar. Pour vinegar into the hot skillet or pan after cooking fish or onions and let it simmer for a few minutes. Boil 1 tablespoon of vinegar in 1 cup of water to eliminate cooking odors from the room.

Corns eliminated from feet. Soak two slices of white bread with 2 slices of onion and 1 cup of vinegar for 24 hours. Place bread on corn, top with a slice of the onion, then wrap with a bandage and leave on overnight. Corns and calluses will fall away, overnight.

Corroded shower and faucet heads cleaned. Unscrew and remove clogged, corroded shower and faucet heads and screens, place in a small container and cover with vinegar. Let soak for several hours or overnight.

COSMETIC VINEGAR FORMULA ONE for bath, hair, and skin. Mix together 2 ounces fresh or 1 ounce each of dried thyme leaves, lavender flowers, spearmint leaves, rosemary leaves, and sage leaves. Steep with 4 cups of apple cider vinegar or wine vinegar for several weeks, then strain. Mix together 1/4 ounce gum camphor, 1/2 ounce gum benzoin, and 3 tablespoons grain alcohol until dissolved. Stir into vinegar, cover, and let stand for three days. Strain, bottle, cap tightly, and label.

COSMETIC VINEGAR FORMULA TWO. Mix together 2 ounces fresh or 1 ounce each of dried orange peel, leaves, and flowers, rose leaves, petals, and hips, willow bark, and chamomile flowers. Steep with 4 cups of apple cider or wine vinegar for several weeks, then strain. Add 1 cup rose water. Bottle, cap tightly, and label.

Cough can be soothed by sprinkling the pillowcase with apple cider vinegar.

Counter tops will shine if wiped down with a mixture of 1 teaspoon liquid soap, 3 tablespoons vinegar, 1/2 teaspoon oil, and 1/2 cup water.

Crayon stains erased. Moisten a soft toothbrush with vinegar and rub out crayon from fabric or other surfaces.

Crystal and glassware rinse. Crystal and glassware will sparkle easily when rinsed in a solution of one part vinegar to three parts warm water.

Cut-flower solution. Keep cut flowers fresh longer by adding 2 tablespoons of vinegar and 1 tablespoon of sugar to each quart of warm water at 100 degrees F.

Dandruff banished and hair made shiny. Rinse after every shampoo with: one-half cup apple cider vinegar mixed into two cups of warm water.

Dandruff. Massage full-strength vinegar into the scalp several times a week before shampooing.

Deodorant stains eliminated. To remove stains from deodorants and antiperspirants, lightly rub fabric with vinegar, then launder as usual.

Digestive problems eased. Peppermint settles and calms the digestive system. Add a couple of teaspoons of peppermint vinegar to a glass of water to ease stomach cramps, diarrhea, or gas. Add a teaspoon of honey and it is one of the best tasting cures for indigestion.

Dish washing solution. 1/2 cup vinegar in dish washing water cuts grease and lets you use less soap.

Disinfectant. Add a splash of vinegar to hot water and use it, with a little soap, to disinfect baby's toys. Be sure to rinse well.

Douche. Although frequent douching is no longer generally recommended, women who are prone to vaginal infections can help prevent them by occasionally douching with a solution of 1 or 2 tablespoons of apple cider vinegar in a quart of warm water.

Drains cleaned out by pouring in 1/2 cup baking soda, followed by 1/2 cup vinegar. In about 10 minutes, run hot water down the drain. Keep drains odor-free by pouring 1/2 cup vinegar down them once a week.

Drains unclogged. Bring vinegar to a boil and pour a small amount down the drain. Let it sit for 5 or 10 minutes, then run hot water. Repeat, if necessary.

Ear infections. Grandmother told us to put diluted vinegar in the ears to ward off infection. Medical authorities now confirm this folk remedy. Head and neck physicians suggest using a mixture of vinegar and alcohol in the ear to prevent "swimmer's ear."

Easter eggs. For bright Easter egg colors, combine 1/2 cup boiling water, 1 teaspoon vinegar, and 1 teaspoon food coloring. Dip eggs until color as desired.

Electric iron cleaned. To remove dark or burned spots on the bottom of an iron, rub with a mixture of vinegar and salt, heat in an aluminum pan, then rise with clean water.

Eyeglasses will clean up and be free of streaks when wiped down with water to which a splash of vinegar has been added.

Fabric color-fast. Immerse fabrics in vinegar before washing.

Fabric creases and thread holes removed. When lengthening a hem, changing a crease, or opening a seam, make a solution of equal parts vinegar and water, then use it to dampen a pressing cloth, pressing as usual.

Fabric dye set. After dyeing fabric, set the color by adding 1 cup of vinegar to the last rinse water.

Faucets and fixtures cleaned with 1/3 cup vinegar and 2/3 cup water. Use it to polish and shine, or brush it into the shower head to remove mineral buildup.

Flavor enhancer. Thyme vinegar is a good addition to meat dishes, as it both flavors and tenderizes. Applied to the body, it acts to deter fungus growth.

Fleas and ticks deterred. Adding a teaspoon of vinegar to each quart of your pet's drinking water acts systematically to deter fleas and ticks.

Floor cleaning. Combine 1/4 cup liquid soap, 1/2 cup vinegar, and 2 gallons of water to make a great floor cleaning solution.

Foot tonic. Walk back and forth in ankle deep bath water to which 1/2 cup apple cider vinegar has been added. Do this for 5 minutes, first thing in the morning, and for 5 minutes before retiring in the evening. Hot, aching feet will feel cooled and soothed.

Freckles. Lighten freckles on the body, not on the face, by rubbing on horseradish vinegar. This is also said to repel mosquitoes.

Frizz from overpermed hair can be solved with a vinegar and water rinse. It also brightens dark hair and adds sparkle to blond hair.

Fruit stains removed from hands. Run hands with vinegar to remove fruit stains.

Furniture dusting. Give furniture a nutty fragrance by cleaning with vinegar to which a little olive oil has been added. When the vinegar evaporates, the wood is left clean and beautiful, with a refreshing fragrance.

Furniture polish can be made from vinegar and lemon oil. Use 3 parts vinegar to 1 part oil for a light weight polish. Use 1 part vinegar to 3 parts oil for a heavy duty polish. An oil and vinegar combination works well for cleaning and polishing. This is because vinegar dissolves and brings up dirt and oil enriches the wood.

Furniture polish. Mix 1/4 cup linseed oil, 1/8 cup vinegar, and 1/8 cup whiskey. Dirt seems to disappear as the alcohol evaporates.

Furniture polish. Wipe furniture with a soft clean cloth moistened with a mixture of 3 tablespoons vinegar and 1 quart water. This also removes cloudy film from varnished surfaces. Rub with grain of the wood. Polish with a soft dry cloth.

Garbage disposal is cleaned and freshened by running a tray of vinegar ice cubes through it once a week. The ice cubes are made with 1/2 cup vinegar poured into the ice tray.

Gargle for sore throat. Just gargle with a glass of warm water to which a tablespoon of apple cider vinegar has been added. Repeat as needed. This also acts as a great mouthwash

Glue can be softened for removal. Simply wet the glued area down with vinegar, or fill a squirt bottle with vinegar and apply to the joint. Keep it wet overnight. Even some of the super glues can be scraped away if they are soaked overnight in vinegar.

Grass and weeds killed. Unwanted grass and weeds along the edge of driveways or between stepping stones meet their demise when you pour vinegar on them.

Hair rinse. After shampooing, rinsing your hair with vinegar leaves it squeaky clean and shining. Vinegar infused with different herbs can enhance different hair colors and condition hair as well. Rosemary and parsley are both good for dark hair, sage darkens graying hair, chamomile brings highlights to blonde or light brown hair, calendula provides conditioning, lavender and lemon verbena add fragrance, linden is good for frequently shampooed hair, and nettles condition hair and control dandruff.

Hairbrushes cleaned by soaking them in 2 cups of hot, soapy water, with 1/2 cup vinegar added to it.

Headache Remedy. Dab an herbal toilet vinegar on your temples while resting. Alternatively, dampen a cloth with some of the vinegar and lay it across your brow.

Headache that will not go away. Try a paper bag hat. Soak the bottom of the open edges of a brown paper bag in apple cider vinegar. Put the bag on the head, just like a chef's hat, and tie it in place with a long scarf. The headache should be relieved in 45 minutes.

Headaches will fade away. Add a dash of apple cider vinegar to the water in a vaporizer and inhale the vapors for 5 minutes. Lay quietly and the headache should be relieved in 20 minutes.

Healthy, richly colored hair can be ensured, well into old age. You need only to start each day with a glass of water to which has been added 4 teaspoons each of apple cider vinegar, black strap molasses, and honey.

Heart disease prevented. Take 1 t. ACV 3 times daily in 1 cup apple cider.

Heavily soiled hands can be cleaned, while giving them a soothing treatment. Simply scrub with cornmeal, moistened with apple cider vinegar. Then rinse in cool water and pat dry.

Herbal hair rinse combinations. With vinegar mix: rosemary, sage, and southernwood leaves or Rosemary and mint leaves or Orange and lemon peels and mint and rosemary leaves or Chamomile and linden flowers and fennel, sage, rosemary, nettle, horsetail, and yarrow leaves.

Hiccups will disappear if you sip, very slowly, a glass of warm water with 1 teaspoon of vinegar in it. Works even better if you sip from the far side of the glass.

Hiccups. Try a small drink of chervil seed vinegar to cure hiccups.

Hose and lingerie life extended. Add vinegar to the rinse water.

Improve light from propane lamps. For more light with less fuel from a propane lamp, remove mantle, place in container, and cover with vinegar. Let soak for several hours. Dry thoroughly before using.

Incontinence. Bathe with soap and water, then wipe the skin with vinegar. This reduces odor and lowers the pH of the skin, which helps prevent the growth of bacteria.

Indigestion. To reduce indigestion, add 2 teaspoons of ACV to a glass of water and drink at each meal.

Infections, as well as plain old itchy ears, are a common complaint of swimmers. Simply dilute vinegar half and half with boiled water then allow to cool. Use to rinse out the ears after each swim. For a more drying solution, mix vinegar half and half with alcohol. This helps to prevent both bacterial and fungal growths.

Ink stains removed from clothes by soaking them in milk for 1 hour. Then cover the stain with a paste of vinegar and cornstarch. When the paste dries, wash the garment as usual.

Ink stains removed. Remove ink marks from fabric by moistening the area with vinegar or by wiping it with a vinegar-dampened clean soft cloth.

Insect and bee stings. Repel insects before going outdoors by rubbing vinegar on your body, particularly the vulnerable wrists, hands, ankles, face, and throat. If bitten, dab apple cider vinegar on bites and stings as soon as possible to draw out the poison and prevent swelling. Thyme vinegar and rosemary vinegar are especially effective for both repelling insects and relieving discomfort from bites.

Insect control and de-worming. Wormwood is quite bitter. This vinegar is best used externally, as a deterrent to fleas and other insects, or applied as a would dressing. For insect control, sprinkle it liberally onto infested areas of rooms.

Intestinal tonic. Dandelion adds its mild laxative nature to vinegar's natural antiseptic qualities. It also has an anti-inflammatory effect on the intestines. This is an old time remedy for ailments of the pancreas and liver, and as such is considered useful in lowering blood pressure. Dandelion is rich in diuretics to pull toxins out of the body.

Iron pans with rust spots can be revitalized. Fill the pan1/4 cup vinegar and water. Boil for 1 hour and wipe the rust away.

Iron without shine. To keep wool and other fabrics from becoming shiny when ironing, place cloth dampened with 1 part vinegar to 2 parts water over the fabric.

Itchy welts and hives, swellings, and blemishes can be eased by the application of a paste made from vinegar and cornstarch. Just pat it on and feel the itch being drawn out as the paste dries.

Keep hiking or camping water fresh. Add several drops of vinegar to a canteen or insulated container of water to keep it fresh longer and make it a better thirst-quencher.

Kitchen work surfaces disinfected and cleaned. Wipe down with full strength white vinegar to clean them and to prevent mold.

Knives sharpened better. When sharpening knives, dampen the whetstone with vinegar.

Laundry rinse water. Get rid of excess suds in either hand or machine washes by adding a cup of vinegar to the rinse water, followed by a clear water rinse.

Laundry soap. 1/4 cup vinegar added to a load of laundry, along with the usual soap, will brighten colors and make whites sparkle. This will also act as a fabric softener, and inhibit mold and fungus growth. Helps to kill athlete's foot germs on socks, too.

Leather furniture polish. Bring 2 cups of linseed oil to a boil for 1 minute, then cool. Stir in 1 cup vinegar. Shake well; apply with a clean soft cloth. Or, mix equal parts of linseed oil and vinegar, shake well, and apply with a clean soft cloth.

Leather shoes preserved and cleaned. Mix together 1 tablespoon vinegar, 1 tablespoon alcohol, 1 teaspoon vegetable oil, and 1/2 teaspoon liquid soap. Wipe it on shoes, then brush until the shoes gleam.

Leg cramps at night can find relief by supplementing meals with a glass of water, fortified with apple cider vinegar.

Leg cramps relieved by combining 1 teaspoon honey, 1 teaspoon apple cider vinegar, and 1 tablespoon calcium lactate in 1/2 glass of water. This is taken once a day.

Lime deposits removed. Tea kettles, coffee brewers, and irons can accumulate lime deposits from hard water. To clean, fill with vinegar and heat or run through one cycle. Rinse well or run through another cycle with plain water before using.

Linens will not yellow. Vinegar in the rinse water of linens, such as tablecloths, napkins, sheets, and pillowcases, keeps them from yellowing in storage.

Liniment. Use one of the herbal cosmetic vinegars as a pleasing alternative to alcohol as a rubbing lotion for aching muscles. Apply to sprains as a hot poultice. Onion slices dipped in vinegar and rubbed on bruises immediately after they occur are said to prevent black-and-blue marks.

Lunch boxes freshened. To make lunch boxes fresh-smelling, dampen a piece of bread with vinegar and leave overnight in the closed box.

Memory can be greatly improved by drinking a glass of warm water before each meal, with a teaspoon of apple cider vinegar stirred in.

Memory problems. Rosemary combines with healthy apple cider vinegar to treat maladies of the head. It boosts the function of mind and memory, relieves tension headaches, and eases dizziness.

Metal cleaner. Combine 2 tablespoons cream of tartar and enough vinegar to make a paste. Rub it on and let it dry. Wash it off with plain warm water and dry with an old towel. Metal will gleam.

Metal primer. Prepare galvanized metal before painting by scouring it with vinegar.

Microwave oven is freshened and cleansed by boiling vinegar water in it. Mix 1/4 cup vinegar and 1 cup water in a small bowl and heat for 5 minutes. This will remove lingering odors and soften baked on food spatters.

Mildew removed. Use vinegar at full strength or mixed with water to remove mildew from clothing, furniture, bathroom fixtures, shower curtains, and so forth.

Mineral buildup on metal can be removed. Just add 1/4 cup to a quart of water for cleaning metal screen and storm doors and aluminum furniture. Add extra vinegar if your water has a particularly high mineral content.

Morning sickness. Upon rising add a teaspoon of apple cider vinegar to a glass of water and drink it.

Mouth healer. Myrrh has long been considered of particular value in maintaining a healthy mouth. Swish this vinegar around in the mouth to hasten healing of sores and to soothe red, swollen gums. This will also sweeten the breath. Ancients used it for treating chest congestion.

Muscles that are tired or sprained can be soothed by wrapping the afflicted area with a cloth wrung out of apple cider vinegar. Leave it on for 3 to 5 minutes and repeat as needed. For extra special relief, add a good dash of cayenne pepper to the vinegar.

Nail polish. Make nail polish more long-lasting by soaking fingertips in a solution of 2 teaspoons vinegar in 1/2 cup warm water for a minute before applying polish.

Nausea or vomiting can be reduced by placing a cloth wrung out of warm apple cider vinegar on the stomach. Replace with another warm cloth when it cools.

New clothes. Add 1/4 cup vinegar to the tub to eliminate manufacturing chemicals and their odors.

New skillets seasoned. To keep foods from sticking in new skillets, first boil some vinegar in pan.

Non-oily stains removed. Remove non-oily, water soluble stains such as wine, perspiration, fruit juice, alcoholic drinks, coffee, tea, soft drinks, salt water, or vomit from carpet, furniture, and fabric by one of several methods. For washable clothing, either dab the area with a clean soft cloth dampened in vinegar or soak the garment in a mixture of 3 parts vinegar to 1 part cool water. For upholstery and carpet, mix 1 or 2 teaspoons each of vinegar and liquid detergent in 2 cups of lukewarm water, then apply the mixture gently with a soft brush or towel. Rinse with clean water, repeating if necessary, then dry by blotting or with a fan or hair dryer.

Old sponges renewed by washing them in vinegar water, then soaking them overnight in 1 quart of water with 1/4 cup vinegar added to it.

Oven cleaned. Apply vinegar at full strength with a sponge to the door and walls.

Paint fumes. Keep a dish or two of vinegar sitting around when painting. The vinegar will absorb the paint odors. For a long painting job, fill a bucket with hay and drizzle 1 cup of vinegar over it. Let this set for 15 minutes. Then add enough water to cover the hay. This will clear the air and keep the room smelling fresh for a couple of days.

Paint on glass removed. Apply heated vinegar to paint on window glass to soften.

Painted surfaces shined and cleaned with 1 tablespoon cornstarch, 1/4 cup vinegar, and 2 cups hot water. Wipe or spray it on and wipe the paint dry immediately. Rub until it shines.

Patent leather cleaned and lustre restored. Wipe with soft cloth moistened with vinegar.

Perspiration odors eliminated. Wipe or rinse article with vinegar.

Perspiration stains in clothes will fade if soaked overnight in 3 gallons of water, to which 1/4 cup vinegar has been added. Use full strength vinegar to remove stains caused by berries, fruits, grass, coffee and tea.

Pet Health. To improve dog's or cat's health, add 1 tablespoon vinegar to pet's water.

Pet or people "potty accidents" cleaned up. Sprinkle vinegar on soiled area, wait a few minutes, then sponge from the center out. Blot with a dry cloth. Repeat, if necessary. Alternatively, combine a small amount of liquid detergent and 3 tablespoons vinegar in 1 quart of warm water. Sponge on soiled area until clean, rinse with a cloth dampened with warm water, then blot with a dry cloth.

Pewter cleaned with a paste made of 1 tablespoon salt, 1 tablespoon flour, and enough vinegar to just barely make the mixture wet. Smear it on discolored pewter and allow to dry. Rub or brush the dried paste off, rinse in hot water, and buff dry.

Pewter cleans up easily if rubbed with cabbage leaves. Just wet the leaves in vinegar and dip them in salt before using them to buff the pewter. Be sure to rinse with cool water and dry thoroughly.

Plastic made anti-static. Vinegar decreases static and attraction of dust on plastic and vinyl. Wipe upholstery with a cloth dampened with a vinegar and water solution. Add a pour of vinegar to rinse water when laundering plastic curtains or tablecloths.

Plastic upholstery cleaned. Wipe plastic or vinyl upholstery with a soft cloth dampened with a solution of water and vinegar.

Poison antidote. Bitter, aromatic rue vinegar was once sprinkled about to ward off contagious diseases and given as an antidote for poison mushrooms and toadstools, as well as the bite of snakes, spiders, and bees.

Pots and pans scoured. Mix equal amounts of flour and salt. Make a paste with vinegar. Rub on pans with a sponge; rinse. Remove normal food stains by soaking pots and pans in full-strength vinegar for 30 minutes, then wash in hot soapy water and rinse.

Produce rinse. Add 1 tablespoon of vinegar per gallon of lukewarm water to remove much of the pesticide residue on fresh fruits and vegetables, plus also killing bugs and germs.

Relieves gas. Spearmint is one of the gentler mints. A bit of spearmint vinegar in a glass of water calms the stomach and digestive system. It also relieves gas and adds a tangy zing to iced tea.

Room odors vanish. Place bowls of vinegar in a room to remove the odors of smoke, paint, vomit, or other substances.

Rust stains removed from fabric. Moisten washable fabric with vinegar, then rub in some salt. Place in sun to dry, then launder as usual.

Rusted, corroded screws and hinges can be loosened. Pour vinegar over the head of a rusty screw or hinge to loosen it. Clean rusty screws, bolts, and nuts by soaking them in vinegar, scrubbing them with a brush, if necessary.

Saddle soap can be made from 1/8 cup liquid soap, 1/8 cup linseed oil, 1/4 cup beeswax, and 1/4 cup vinegar. Warm the beeswax, slowly, in the vinegar. Then add the soap and oil. Keep the mixture warm until it will all mix together smoothly. Then cool until it is solid. Rub it onto good leather, then buff to a high shine.

Salt marks on leather removed. Wipe salt-stained boots or shoes with a soft clean cloth moistened with vinegar.

Scorch marks dissolved. With soft clean cloth dampened with vinegar, lightly rub scorched fabric. Wipe with clean cloth. Not effective on heavily scorched items.

Seed starting. To improve germination of woody-coated seeds, such as asparagus, okra, and sweet peas, rub seeds between two sheets of coarse sandpaper, then soak overnight in a pint of warm water with 1/2 cup of vinegar and a squirt of liquid soap. Use water treatment without sandpaper for nasturtium, parsley, parsnip, and beet seeds.

Sharp creases while ironing clothes. Dampen fabric with cloth moistened with solution of 1 part vinegar to 2 parts water. Place heavy brown paper over the crease and press.

Shower curtains cleaned. To remove mildew and soap scum from plastic shower curtains, launder the curtain with a bath towel in the washing machine, adding a cup of vinegar during the rinse cycle.

Silk rinse. After hand-washing silk clothing in mild soap, remove soap residue by adding a capful of vinegar to clean, cool rinse water. Roll in towel to remove excess water; hang to dry until slightly damp. Press on wrong side with dry iron.

Sinusitis and facial neuralgia. Relieve the pain of sinusitis and facial neuralgia by drinking a glass of water with 1 teaspoon of apple cider vinegar added every hour for seven doses.

Skin is made soft, radiant and blemish-free by conditioning the skin while sleeping with a covering of strawberries and vinegar. Mash 3 large strawberries into 1/4 cup vinegar and let it sit for 2 hours. Then strain the vinegar through a cloth. Pat the strawberry-flavored vinegar onto the face and neck. Wash off in the morning. Skin will soon be free of pimples and blackheads.

Skin protected from the ravages of the summer sun by applying a protective lotion of olive oil and apple cider vinegar. Mixed half and half, this combination helps prevent sunburn and chapping.

Soap scum removal. Dilute ACV half and half with water and use it to rub down your body after bathing. It will leave your skin naturally soft, pH balanced, and free of soapy film. It also acts as a natural deodorant.

Soft leather is softened and cleaned with a vitamin enriched solution. Heat 1/2 cup vinegar to the boiling point. Drop in 3 vitamin E capsules and let stand, undisturbed, until the capsules dissolve. Add 1/2 cup lemon or olive oil and blend well.

Soften blankets and sweaters. Add 2 cups of vinegar to rinse water to remove soap odor and make material soft and fluffy.

Sore throat and fevers. Enhance the healing properties of chicken soup by adding 1 tablespoon vinegar, 1 crushed garlic clove, and a few drops of hot pepper sauce to a cup of hot chicken broth. Or, simply mix 1 tablespoon each of honey and apple cider vinegar or 2 tablespoons of sweetened raspberry or blackberry vinegar in a cup of hot water to promote rest, soothe a scratchy throat, and relieve congestion.

Sore throat discomfort is eased and healing accelerated by sipping occasionally on a syrup made of 1/2 cup apple cider vinegar, 1/2 cup water, 1 teaspoon cayenne pepper, and 3 tablespoons honey.

Sore throat. Ease the discomfort of a sore throat and speed healing by sipping occasionally on a syrup made of 1/2 cup apple cider vinegar, 1/2 cup water, 1 teaspoon cayenne pepper, and 3 tablespoons honey.

Sore throat. To relieve the pain of a sore throat caused by a cold, mix together 1/4 cup honey and 1/4 cup apple cider vinegar. Take 1 tablespoon every 4 hours. May be taken more often if needed.

Stainless steel cleans up nicely if scrubbed with baking soda which has been dampened with just a little vinegar. Or just moisten a soft cloth with vinegar and polish.

Stains on wood lifted. To remove dark stains from wood floors or furniture, first clean the area with coarse steel wool dipped in mineral spirits. Next, scrub the stain with vinegar, allowing it to penetrate for several minutes. Repeat, if necessary, then rise with water and wax.

Static cling and lint can be reduced with a vinegar rinse. Some laundry stains can be soaked out in equal parts of milk and vinegar.

Stickers, decals, and glue removed. Apply vinegar directly or with a clean soft cloth to remove price tags, bumper stickers, decals, or glue.

Stuck-on food should be soaked or simmered in 2 cups of water and 1/2 cup of vinegar. The food will soften and lift off in a few minutes.

Tenderizer and flavor enhancer. Sage vinegar not only adds its delicate hint of flavoring to meats, it tenderizes them. Splashed into soups and dressings, it serves up a tranquilizer for frazzled nerves.

Toilet cleaner can be made from 1 cup borax and 1 cup vinegar. Pour the vinegar all over the stained area of the toilet, then sprinkle the borax over the vinegar. Allow it all to soak for 2 hours, then simply brush and flush.

Toothache. Rub calendula or acacia vinegar for temporary relief.

Unsettled stomach will calm down if you sip quietly on a glass of very warm water, to which has been added 1 tablespoon honey and 1 tablespoon vinegar. This is also good for easing gas.

Urinary tract. A small amount of vinegar, taken every day, keeps the urinary tract nice and acidic. This is useful to reduce the likelihood of getting a kidney or bladder infection.

Urine neutralized. When urine leaks onto delicate skin surfaces, it can irritate or even burn sensitive skin. Vinegar compresses, applied to the skin, help restore its natural condition, neutralize leaking urine, and promote healing.

Varicose veins relieved by wrapping the legs with a cloth wrung out of apple cider vinegar. Leave this on, with the legs propped up, for 30 minutes, morning and evening. Considerable relief will be noticed within 6 weeks. To speed up the healing process, follow each treatment with a glass of warm water, to which a teaspoon of apple cider vinegar has been added. Sip slowly, and add a teaspoon of honey if feeling fatigued.

Vinegar painting. Decorate finished or unfinished wooden picture frames, furniture, or other objects with a texturizing tool and a vinegar-paint solution. To make the paint, mix 1/2 cup white vinegar, 1 teaspoon granulated sugar, and a squeeze of clear liquid dish detergent. In a second container, place 2 tablespoons of dry powdered poster paint and add enough vinegar solution to make a mixture that doesn't run when brushed on a vertical surface. Brush the solution on the surface, and then use a texturing tool, such as a comb, a feather, a crumbled paper, or a sponge, to create the desired effect. When done, let the paint dry thoroughly, then apply several coats of clear polyurethane.

Vinyl surfaces are best cleaned with 1/2 cup vinegar, 2 teaspoons liquid soap, and 1/2 cup water. Use a soft cloth to wipe this mixture onto vinyl furniture, then rinse with clear water and buff dry.

Walls, woodwork, and blinds cleaned. Mix 1 cup ammonia, 1/2 cup vinegar, and 1/4 cup baking soda in 1 gallon warm water. Apply with sponge or soft cloth; then rinse.

Water rings eliminated from wooden furniture. Combine vinegar and olive oil in equal parts. On a clean, soft cloth, work mixture with the grain to erase water rings.

Water scale build up on glass shower doors can be removed with alum and vinegar. Mix 1 teaspoon alum into 1/4 cup vinegar. Wipe it on the glass and scrub with a soft brush. Rinse with lots of water and buff until completely dry. Alum is aluminum sulfate.

Water spots. A splash of vinegar added to rinse water will keep glasses from water spotting. It kills germs, too.

Weight loss. Drink a glass of warm water, with a single teaspoon of apple cider vinegar stirred in, before each meal. It moderates the appetite and melts away fat.

Window cleaner. Combine 1/2 teaspoon liquid soap, 1/4 cup vinegar, and 2 cups water. Soak a sponge or small cloth in this mixture, then wring it out. Store the window cloth in a glass jar with a tight fitting lid until needed. Then simply wipe spots and smears from dirty windows. They will clean up easily without streaks.

Window cleaner. Just mix 1/4 cup vinegar into 1 quart water and put it in a spray bottle. Spray it onto windows and wipe off immediately with clean, soft cloth.

Windows and mirrors. Several variations of window cleaner can be made at home. 1) Mix 1 tablespoon of vinegar in 1 quart of water. 2) Mix 1 to 2 tablespoons of vinegar and 3 to 8 tablespoons of ammonia in 1 quart of water. 3) Mix 1/4 cup each of vinegar and ammonia with 1 tablespoon of cornstarch in 1 quart of water.

Windshields frost-free. Wipe windshields with a sponge soaked in a solution of three parts vinegar to one part water to prevent frost from forming on them.

Wine and catsup stains removed from washable cotton polyester and blends. Sponge with vinegar within 24 hours. Launder as usual.

Wood cutting blocks. Once a week, rub them with baking soda. They spray on full strength vinegar. Let sit for 5 minutes, then rinse in clear water. It will bubble and froth as these two natural chemicals interact.

Wood scratches can be repaired with vinegar and iodine. Mix equal parts of each in a small dish and apply with an artist's paint brush. Add extra iodine for a deeper color, more vinegar for a lighter color.

Woodworm deterred in furniture. Combine 5 ounces linseed oil, 5 ounces turpentine, 2 ounces vinegar, and 2 ounces denatured alcohol. Shake well, apply with a soft clean cloth to wood furniture.

Wrapping tape adheres better. Add a few drops of vinegar to the water used to moisten wrapping tape.

[1]. Kaufman, MB, Pediatric Emergency Care, vol.8, no.1, p.27, Feb.1992

[2]. Brighenti, F., et al., European Journal of Clinical Nutrition, vol.49, no.4, p.242, Apr.1995

[3]. Whiting, SJ, et al., Journal of the American College of Nutrition, vol.11, no.5, p.553, Oct.1992

[4]. Ghebrekidan, H, Ethiopian Medical Journal, vol.30, no.1, p.23, Jan.1992

Chapter 7

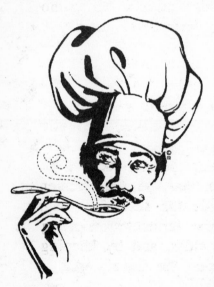

VINEGAR RECIPES

nutritious and delicious ways to use more
vinegar in your diet

The secret to success in life is to eat what you want and let the food fight it out inside. Mark Twain, a.k.a. Samuel Clemens

✿ PERSONAL PROFILE. WR was a bright happy, healthy child and had as much energy as any 8 year old boy. Except WR had a secret. He was a bedwetter. He had some friends, but never hosted or attended any overnight parties due to his embarrassment at wetting the bed. WR's mother asked me for help. We found that WR had extremely active kidneys, though the medical test showed that his kidneys were functioning well. Sometimes frequent urination is caused by the body's attempts to bring the pH of the blood into balance. Vinegar can often correct this imbalance. We gave WR a glass of apple cider with 1 teaspoon of apple cider vinegar each morning and evening with his meal. For 3 hours before bedtime, he was instructed to avoid any fluid intake. At bedtime, he took a tablespoon of raw honey, for its ability to bind water. And after each time that he urinated, WR exercised the same muscles that hold the urine back, by squeezing that sphincter muscle for isometrics of 10 seconds each for 5 sets. Within 2 weeks, WR ceased wetting the bed permanently. He found a new identity and became more active with his friends. While bedwetting is not a serious or fatal flaw, it can be disastrous on a young person's self-image. In this case, vinegar and honey cured the problem.

Vinegar is one of the most versatile, tasty, and healthy additions to any kitchen. Because of its acid content, vinegar is able to tenderize meats, add tartness to flavors, curdle milk, and preserve foods from bacterial infection. Don't miss a day without using vinegar somewhere in your diet. Bon appetit!!

MAKING VINEGAR

Vinegar making requires two separate, distinct fermentations. The first, called alcoholic (or vinous) changes natural sugars to alcohol. The second, called acid (or acetic) changes alcohol to acetic acid. It is important that the first fermenting be completely finished before the second is begun.

You can hurry the first fermentation along by adding a little yeast to the cider, and by keeping it warm. At around 80 degrees, the liquids will convert very fast.

To speed up the second fermentation, add a little mother-of-vinegar to the mix. The more air the mixture gets during this second part of the process, the faster it will convert to vinegar.

Caution: Mother-of-vinegar must not get into the liquid until practically all the sugar has been converted to alcohol.

The vinegar bacterium is present wherever there is air. This is why any wine which is spilled at a winery must be mopped up at once. Bacterial could get started in the wine and sour it all! If a winery makes both wine and vinegar, separate rooms are used for each. Barrels from vinegar making are never used for storing wine.

AN OLD APPLE CIDER VINEGAR RECIPE

Put cut up apples in a stone crock and cover them with warm water. Tie a cheesecloth over the top and set in a warm place for 4-6 months. Then strain off the vinegar. For faster action, add a lump of raw bread dough to the crock.

Let this sweet apple cider stand open in a jug for 4-6 weeks and it will become vinegar.

Place apple and peach peelings, and a handful of grape skins, in a wide mouthed jar and cover these fruit leavings with cold water. Set in a warm place and add a couple of fresh apple cores every few days. When a scum forms on top, stop adding fresh fruit and let it thicken. When the vinegar is good and strong, strain it through a cheesecloth.

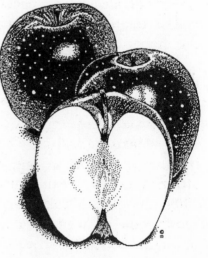

Make vinegar in a special hurry by adding brown sugar, molasses, or yeast to cider.

OTHER VINEGAR RECIPES

Because the sugar content of honey varies a lot, you may want to check and see if your water to honey ratio is correct. Do this by dropping an egg into the mixture. It should float in the liquid, with only a small spot showing above the surface. If the egg sinks, add more honey. If the egg floats too high, add more water. This method should assure you that the specific gravity of the mix is about 1.05, which is ideal for making good honey vinegar.

Dandelions add a unique taste to honey vinegar. Just add 3 cups of blossoms to the honey and water. Be sure to strain it before using!

Dark, strong flavored honeys will ferment much faster than light, mild ones. Add a cup or two of fruit juice or molasses to the honey to speed up the change to vinegar.

For an extra special, clover-flavored, vinegar add a quart of freshly washed clover blossoms to the honey and water mix.

Let a bottle of wine stand, open to the air, in the summer sun. In about 2 weeks it will turn into a nice vinegar. Make winter vinegar by letting wine stand open to the air for about a month.

Make a deeply colored honey vinegar by pouring 1 gallon boiling water over 5 pounds of strained honey. Stir until all the honey is melted. Then dissolve 1 cake (or package) of yeast in 1 tablespoon of warm water. Spread the yeast on a dry corn cob or a slice of toast and float it on the top of the honey-water. Cover the container with a cloth and let it set for 16 days. Take out the corn cob, skim off the scum, and strain the liquid. Now let it stand for a month or so, until it turns into vinegar.

Put 2 pounds of raisins in a gallon of water and set it in a warm place. In 2 months it will become white wine vinegar. Just strain the vinegar off and bottle it. Make some more vinegar by adding another 1/2 pound of raisins to the dredges and going through the process again.

Raspberry vinegar can be prepared by pouring 2 quarts of water over 1 quart of freshly washed red or black raspberries. Cover lightly and let stand overnight. Strain off the liquid and discard the berries. Now prepare 1 more quart of fresh raspberries and pour the same liquid over them. Let this set overnight. Do this for a total of 5 times. Then add 1 pound of sugar to the liquid and stir until it is dissolved. Set the mixture aside, uncovered, for a couple of months. Strain before using.

SPICY VINEGAR
1 quart vinegar
1/2 cup sugar
1 tablespoon cinnamon
1 teaspoon allspice
1 tablespoon mustard
1 teaspoon cloves
1 teaspoon salt
4 tablespoons grated horseradish
2 tablespoons celery seed

Combine all ingredients and bring to a boil. Pour over pickles or sliced, cooked beets.

HOT PEPPER VINEGAR

Add 1/2 ounce cayenne pepper to 1 pint of vinegar. Shake every other day for 2 weeks. Strain before using.

CELERY VINEGAR

1 teaspoon salt
2 cups chopped celery
1 quart vinegar

Boil for 3 minutes and seal it all in a glass jar for 3 weeks. Strain and use.

CHILI VINEGAR

Add 3 ounces chopped chilies to a quart of vinegar. Cap for 2 weeks and strain. For a super hot vinegar, increase steeping time.

CUCUMBER-ONION VINEGAR

Slice very thin, 2 pickling cucumbers and 1 small onion. Add 1 pint boiling vinegar, 1 teaspoon salt and a dash of white pepper. Seal into a glass jar for 5 weeks and then strain. Allow sediment to settle and pour into a clean bottle and cap. Onion may be left out for a light vinegar that is especially good on fruit.

HORSERADISH VINEGAR

Grate 1/4 cup horseradish into a quart of boiling vinegar. Seal for 3 days and then strain out the horseradish. Or prepare an easy vinegar by simply putting a few large pieces of fresh horseradish in a bottle of vinegar. After 2 weeks, begin using the vinegar, without removing the horseradish. It will increase in strength over time.

ONION VINEGAR

Peel three small onions and drop them, whole, into 1 quart vinegar. Wait 3 weeks. Remove the onions and use the vinegar, very sparingly. A few drops will be enough to season most foods.

NASTURTIUM VINEGAR

1 quart nasturtium flowers
2 cloves garlic
1 quart vinegar

Combine and age for 6 weeks. Strain and use. May be improved by adding 2 peeled cloves of garlic.

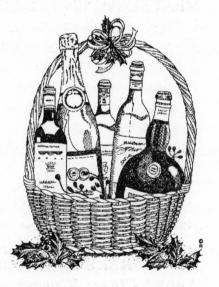

HERB TEA VINEGAR

Add 1/2 cup of strong herb tea to a quart of vinegar.

TARRAGON VINEGAR

Put 1/4 cup tarragon leaves in a pint bottle of vinegar and let set for 8 weeks. Use on cooked and raw vegetables.

GARLIC VINEGAR

Separate and peel all the cloves of a large garlic bulb. Put them in a quart of vinegar and allow to steep for 2 weeks. Strain off the vinegar and discard the garlic. Only a few drops are needed in most dishes.

MINT VINEGAR

Stuff a bottle full of mint leaves. Then fill the bottle with hot vinegar, cap and let set for 6 weeks. Strain and use with meats or in cool drinks.

MEAT FLAVORING VINEGAR

1 large grated onion
3 red peppers, chopped fine
2 tablespoons brown sugar
1 tablespoon celery seed
1 tablespoon dry mustard
1 teaspoon turmeric
1 teaspoon pepper
1/2 teaspoon salt

Stir all ingredients into a quart of vinegar. Let age for 3 weeks. 2 tablespoons of this will flavor and color a stew or gravy.

HERB VINEGAR COMBINATIONS
Apple Cider Vinegar with:
Champagne Vinegar with:
Dill, bay, and garlic
Dill, mustard seeds, lemon balm, and garlic
Garlic, basil, whole cracked nutmeg, and whole cloves
Horseradish, shallot, and hot red pepper
Lemon balm, lemon verbena, lemon thyme, lemongrass, and lemon zest
Tarragon, chives, lemon balm, shallots, and garlic

Malt Vinegar with:
Tarragon, Garlic chives, whole cloves, and garlic or shallot

Red Wine Vinegar with:
Basil, mint, tarragon, rosemary, sage, garlic, fresh ginger root, bay, green onions, and whole allspice berries, cloves, mustard seeds, cumin seeds, black peppercorns, and cinnamon stick

Basil, oregano, garlic, and black peppercorns

Basil, rosemary, tarragon, marjoram, mint, bay, dill seed, black peppercorns, and whole allspice berries and cloves

Burnet, borage, and dill

Cilantro, garlic, and fresh ginger root

Cilantro, hot red pepper, and garlic

Cilantro, sage, rosemary, bay, and hot red pepper

Garlic, jalapeno peppers, and black peppercorns

Lemon thyme, rosemary, and black peppercorns

Lemongrass, lemon verbana, lemon zest, and green peppercorns

Marjoram, basil, mint, dill, rosemary, bay, and whole allspice berries, black peppercorns, and cloves

Marjoram, burnet, and lemon balm

Mint, rosemary, bay, sage, tarragon, garlic, and whole cloves, cinnamon stick, black peppercorns, allspice berries, and mustard seed

Rosemary, savory, sage, basil, bay, and garlic

Sage, parsley, and shallots

Thyme, rosemary, hyssop, fennel, oregano, and garlic

Thyme, rosemary, oregano, and basil

Sherry Vinegar with:
Basil, rosemary, tarragon, dill, sorrel, mint, chives, and garlic
Parsley, thyme, rosemary, and bay
Rosemary, oregano, sage, basil, parsley, garlic, and black peppercorns
Sage, whole allspice berries, cloves, and cinnamon stick
Shallot, thyme, and bay
White Wine Vinegar with:
Basil, chives, garlic chives, tarragon, borage, and burnet
Basil, parsley, fennel, and garlic
Borage, dill, and shallots
Dill, basil, tarragon, and lemon balm
Dill, mint, and garlic cloves
Marjoram, burnet, thyme, tarragon, parsley, and chives
Mint and cardamom seeds
Mint, lemon balm, and lemon basil
Orange mint and orange zest
Orange mint, coriander seeds, garlic, and orange zest
Oregano, cilantro, garlic, and hot red pepper
Parsley, lovage, chervil, savory, thyme, rosemary, tarragon, shallots, and black peppercorns
Rosemary, thyme, marjoram, savory, lavender, bay, garlic, and hot red pepper
Savory, tarragon, chervil, basil, and chives
Tarragon, anise hyssop, hyssop, and lemon balm
Tarragon, chervil, borage, watercress, garlic, and hot red pepper

Tarragon, elder flowers, spearmint, lemon balm, shallot, garlic, and whole cloves and peppercorns
Tarragon, lemon thyme, and chive blossoms
Thai basil and hot red pepper

SPECIAL VINEGARS

BLACKBERRY VINEGAR
4 pounds fresh blackberries
Enough malt vinegar to cover blackberries
3/4 pound honey for every pint extracted blackberry juice

Wash the blackberries in cold running water. Place in a glass, earthenware or ceramic pot. Cover with malt vinegar for three days. Stir once a day. Strain through a sieve and drain thoroughly by placing a plate on top and putting a weight on the plate. let it drip all day. Measure the juice and allow 3/4 pound of honey per pint of juice. Simmer in another glass, ceramic or earthenware pot for five minutes. Collect and discard the top scum. Let cool, then bottle, cork and label.

It is reported that this vinegar is excellent for fevers, arthritis and gout. The dosage here is 1 Tbs dissolved in a large cup of distilled water. Use three times a day. This preparation will somewhat ease the pain and is said to eventually help dissolve arthritic deposits. This vinegar is also good for anemia and has helped many heart patients.

ANTI-EPIDEMIC VINEGAR
1 quart apple cider vinegar
1 pound garlic buds for 8 oz juice

8 oz comfrey root
4 oz oak bark
4 oz marshmallow root
4 oz mullein flowers
4 oz rosemary flowers
4 oz lavender flowers
4 oz wormwood
4 oz black walnut leaves
12 oz glycerin

Make separate teas of each of the herbs. First soak each ounce of herb in clean spring water. After about half a day, simmer each herb separately for 10 minutes. Steep for half an hour. Strain out, simmer again, and reduce each herb so that it is concentrated. Press garlic buds into 8 oz of concentrated juice. Add 12 oz of glycerin to preserve it. Place in a large bottle. Label. Close. You may want to add paraffin for additional preservation power.

Dosage: 1-3 tsp during epidemics, or 1 tsp per hour if someone in the family is ill with a communicable disease. Dilute with water if too strong to the taste, or add to hot herbal tea.

BEAUTY VINEGARS

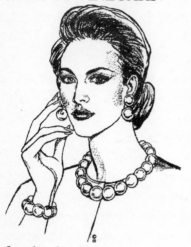

Here are three excellent herb vinegar recipes. You can use them as a refreshing, aromatic addition to bathwater or as an invigorating facial splash. They also make delightful dressings for salad.

One

1 qt apple cider vinegar
2 Tbs dried herbs (or 2 Tbs fresh herbs)

Place vinegar in a ceramic or glass pot. Bring to a brief boil. Turn off heat. Add herbs. Pour into vinegar jar. Use leftover vinegar for body wash or addition to bath.

Two

1 qt apple cider vinegar
1 handful fresh mint or tarragon (or 3 Tbs dried mint)

Wash mint, bruise leaves well and pack into jar. Cover tightly and let stand two weeks. Strain out the herbs. (If dried mint is used, first simmer the vinegar, bring to a boil, and then pour over the mint.)

Three

1/2 pint apple cider vinegar
1 oz rose petals
1/2 pint rosewater
1/2 pint vinegar

1 oz several different kinds of aromatic flowers, such as lavender, sweet violet, rosemary

Mix and steep for two weeks.

VINEGAR OF THE GARDEN

2 qts apple cider vinegar
2 Tbs lavender
2 Tbs rosemary
2 Tbs sage
2 Tbs wormwood
2 Tbs rue
2 Tbs mint
2 Tbs garlic buds

Combine the dried herbs, except the garlic, and steep in the vinegar in the sun for two weeks. Strain and rebottle. Label. Add several cloves of garlic. Close lid. When garlic has steeped for several days, strain out. Melt paraffin wax around the lid to preserve the contents, or add 4 oz of glycerin for preservation.

TIPS FOR USING VINEGAR IN THE KITCHEN

Bean soups, pasta or bean salads get a robust flavor by replacing salt with vinegar.

Boiled beef. Improve the taste and texture of boiled beef by adding 1 or more tablespoons of vinegar to the cooking oil.

Boiled ham. Improve the flavor of boiled ham by adding vinegar to the cooking water.

Buttermilk substitute. To substitute for buttermilk in a recipe, add 1 tablespoon vinegar to a cup of fresh or canned evaporated milk, then let it stand for 5 minutes.

Cellulose can be broken down with vinegar, so use it on coarse, fibrous, or stingy cooked vegetables such as beets, cabbage, spinach, lettuce, and celery. Sprinkle it on raw vegetables such as cucumbers, kale, lettuce, carrots, and broccoli.

Clean fruits and vegetables. Wash fruits and vegetables in water with vinegar added to remove pesticides, heavy metal residues, and insects. Use 2 1/2 tablespoons of vinegar to a gallon of water.

Cleaning fish. Before scaling fish, rub with vinegar to make scaling easier and keep hands from smelling fishy.

Desserts. Add a teaspoon of vinegar to pies and other desserts to enhance flavor and reduce cloying sweetness.

Fish. Add a tablespoon of more of vinegar to fried or boiled fish when cooking. To keep fish white, soak the fish for 20 minutes in a mixture of 1 quart water and 2 tablespoons vinegar.

Fried foods. Make fried foods seem less greasy by adding a tablespoon of vinegar to the deep fryer or skillet before adding the oil.

Fruits and vegetables. Keep potatoes from turning black or apples and avocados from browning by tossing cut up pieces with vinegar or adding one or two teaspoons of vinegar to the cooking water or water they're kept in until ready for use in recipes.

Garlic substitute. Use garlic wine vinegar in place of fresh garlic in any recipe. A teaspoon is the equivalent of a small clove of garlic.

Gelatin. To keep gelatin firmer in warm weather, add a teaspoon of vinegar.

Ginger fresh. Peel ginger and grate or process in a food processor. Fill a clean jar and cover with sherry or balsamic vinegar. Store in refrigerator.

Hamburgers. Add a teaspoon of garlic wine vinegar and 1/2 teaspoon mustard to a pound of hamburger.

Hard boiled eggs. Eggs that are cracked can be hard-cooked without the white running out by adding vinegar to the boiling water.

Homemade bread. Add a sheen to the crust of homemade bread by brushing the top of bread with vinegar several minutes before done, then returning it to the oven to complete baking.

Mashed potatoes. After the last of the hot milk has been added to mashed potatoes, add a teaspoon of vinegar and beat them a little more.

Mayonnaise retrieval. Get the last remaining contents of mayonnaise or salad dressing out of the jars by adding a bit of vinegar and shaking.

Meringue. Make fluffier, more stable meringue by adding vinegar in the proportion of 1/2 teaspoon of vinegar to three egg whites.

Mold on cheese. Keep cheese soft and mold-free by wrapping it in a cloth saturated with vinegar, then storing it in an airtight container in the refrigerator.

Mold-less canning jars. To prevent mold on the outside of canning jars, wipe jars with vinegar after they are sealed.

Muscle fiber in meat is tenderized by the acid in vinegar. It also works on fish such as salmon, and on lobster, oysters, fruits, and vegetables. Therefore, less expensive cuts of meat can be used in most recipes. They are healthier, since these are the cuts with the least fat.

Pimiento peppers. An opened jar of canned pimiento peppers can be kept for weeks if they are covered with vinegar and refrigerated.

Poached eggs. To poach eggs, put a saucepan of water on medium-high heat, add 2 teaspoons of vinegar, and bring to a simmer. Crack an egg into a cup. With a wooden spoon, briskly stir the water, creating a whirlpool. Pour the egg into the vortex. Cook for 2 minutes.

Revive wilted vegetables. Freshen vegetables that are slightly wilted in a cold water-vinegar solution.

Rising bread. To help bread rise, add 1 tablespoon of vinegar for every 2 1/2 cups flour when adding other liquids, reducing those liquids accordingly. This makes the gluten more elastic.

Salvage over-salted food. Food that has been oversalted can be rescued by adding a teaspoon each of vinegar and sugar, then reheating.

Seven-minute frosting. To keep seven-minute frosting white and soft, add 1/2 teaspoon vinegar to a recipe calling for 1 1/2 cups sugar and 2 egg whites.

Soups and tomato sauce. One or two tablespoons of vinegar added to soups or tomato sauces in the last five minutes of cooking enhances their flavors.

Steamed vegetables. Retain bright color and vitamin content of vegetables by adding 2 teaspoons of vinegar to the water for steaming. This also prevents off-odors.

Store herbs. Instead of drying herbs, try storing them in vinegar. Loosely pack a scaled jar with fresh herbs, add warmed vinegar to cover by one inch, making sure all leaves are immersed, then cover tightly. Herbs can be stored at room temperature and used in the same proportion as dried herbs. This works especially well with tarragon and white wine vinegar.

Tenderize meats. Marinate meats in a herb-flavored wine vinegar to tenderize them. The sourness cooks away, leaving the flavor of the herbs and wine.
The same technique also makes strudel dough more pliant.

Unless directions indicate otherwise, all flavored vinegars are made by adding flavoring agents to apple cider vinegar and allowing it to age.

Vinegar for wine. When a recipe calls for wine, substitute vinegar, diluting one part of vinegar with three parts of water.

Wild game. To remove the gamey flavor from wild meat, soak the meat in a vinegar-water solution before cooking.

RECIPES

Substitute any of your favorite flavored vinegers to the recipes.

Sauces

BASIC MARINADE
This tenderizes and flavors meat
1/2 cup vinegar
2 cups wine or meat broth
1 medium onion, grated
2 cloves garlic, crushed
1 tablespoon Worcestershire sauce
1 tablespoon mustard (dry or prepared)
2 whole cloves
1 bay leaf
1 tablespoon mixed dry herbs of rosemary & oregano
1 tablespoon soy sauce
    Combine all ingredients. Pour over meat; refrigerate 24 hours or longer. Turn meat occasionally. When ready to cook meat, strain marinade if necessary, and use some of it as all or part of the liquid in cooking the meat. Fine for stews, pot roasts. Makes about 2 1/2 cups marinade.

MEXICAN MARINADE
3/4 cup onion, minced
3/4 cup vinegar

1/3 cup fresh hot green pepper, cored, seeded, and minced
3 tablespoons fresh cilantro, minced
3 cloves garlic, minced
1 teaspoon salt
Combine all ingredients in a glass or ceramic dish.

COFFEE-MOLASSES MARINADE
1 cup strong coffee
1/2 cup garlic vinegar
1/4 cup unsulfured molasses
1/4 cup Dijon mustard
1 tablespoon Worcestershire sauce
In a small heavy nonreactive saucepan, combine all ingredients and bring to a boil over medium heat. Reduce heat to low and simmer for 2 minutes. Cool before transferring to a glass or ceramic dish.

SOY SAUCE MARINADE
1/3 cup soy sauce
1/2 cup canola oil
1/3 cup vinegar
1/4 cup dry sherry (opt.)
1/4 cup honey
1/4 cup green onion, thinly sliced
2 tablespoons tomato paste
1 tablespoon fresh ginger, minced
2 cloves garlic, minced
1 teaspoon hot red pepper sauce
Combine all ingredients in a heavy nonreactive saucepan and bring to a boil over

medium heat. Reduce heat and simmer for 5 minutes. Cool and transfer to a glass or ceramic dish.

FRESH TOMATO SAUCE
Serve over pasta or grilled fish or chicken.
2 cups tomatoes, peeled, seeded, and chopped
1/4 cup vinegar
1/2 cup fresh parsley, minced
2 tablespoons fresh basil, minced
2 tablespoons fresh spearmint, minced
2 cloves garlic, minced
1 teaspoon salt
1/2 teaspoon freshly ground black pepper
1/2 cup olive oil

In large nonreactive bowl, combine all ingredients except olive oil. Add oil in a thin stream, whisking continually until it is well combined. Serve at room temperature.

Salads

AVOCADO DRESSING
1/4 cup olive oil
1/4 cup vinegar
1 avocado, peeled and pitted
1/4 cup green onion, thinly sliced
1 tablespoon fresh dill, minced
1 tablespoon fresh celery leaves, minced
1 teaspoon fresh tarragon, minced
Salt and freshly ground black pepper to taste

Combine all ingredients in a blender and process until smooth. Cover and chill for several hours.

GINGER DRESSING
1/3 cup olive oil
1 tablespoon chopped ginger
1/3 cup vinegar
2 tablespoons soy sauce
2 tablespoons honey
2 tablespoons fresh lemon juice
1 tablespoon Dijon mustard
1 teaspoon untoasted sesame oil
1 small hot red pepper
In a small heavy nonreactive saucepan, combine all ingredients. Bring to a boil over medium heat, reduce heat to low, and simmer for 3 minutes. Remove hot pepper. Pour over greens while still hot.

VINAIGRETTE
1/2 teaspoon salt
1/2 teaspoon paprika
1/8 teaspoon pepper
3/4 cup apple cider vinegar
1/2 cup olive oil
1 tablespoon minced pickles
1 tablespoon grated green pepper
1 tablespoon chopped parsley
1 tablespoon dry mustard
1 tablespoon sugar
1 tablespoon tarragon vinegar

Mix well and chill the vinaigrette. Serve with cold meats or heat it and pour over broccoli, artichokes, or asparagus.

HOT POTATO SALAD
4 medium potatoes
4 slices turkey bacon
1/4 cup chopped onion
1/2 teaspoon salt
1/4 teaspoon pepper
3 tablespoons vinegar
2 tablespoons white wine
2 teaspoons sugar
2 hard-cooked eggs, chopped
Boil potatoes in jackets until tender. Peel and dice, but keep hot. Fry bacon until crisp, drain and crumble. Sauté onions lightly, add salt, pepper, vinegar, wine and sugar. Heat, then pour over hot potatoes. Add chopped hard-cooked eggs, and mix to blend dressing through salad. Serve immediately.

BLACK BEAN SALAD
Two 16-ounce cans black beans, drained and rinsed
1 cup cherry tomatoes, stemmed and quartered
1/2 cup green onions, thinly sliced
1/2 cup corn, cooked
1/2 cup sweet red pepper, cored, seeded, and diced
1/2 cup sweet yellow pepper, cored, seeded, and diced
2 tablespoons jalapeno pepper, cored, seeded, and diced
1/4 cup fresh cilantro, minced

1/4 cup vinegar
2 tablespoons olive oil
2 tablespoons dry sherry (opt.)
1 tablespoon fresh marjoram, minced
1 teaspoon coarse-grain mustard
1/2 teaspoon ground cumin seeds
1/2 teaspoon hot red pepper sauce
Salt and freshly ground black pepper to taste
   In a large nonreactive bowl, combine beans, cherry tomatoes, green onions, corn, red and yellow sweet peppers, jalapeno peppers, and cilantro. In a small glass bowl, whisk together the vinegar, olive oil, sherry, marjoram, mustard, cumin, hot pepper sauce, salt, and pepper. Pour over the bean mixture and toss until all ingredients are coated. Cover and refrigerate for several hours before serving to allow flavors to blend.

BARLEY SALAD
1 1/2 cups barley, cooked
1/3 cup sweet green pepper, cored, seeded, and diced
1/3 cup sweet red pepper, cored, seeded, and diced
1 cup corn, cooked
1/4 cup vinegar
3 tablespoons olive oil
2 tablespoons fresh basil, minced
2 tablespoons fresh parsley, minced
1/4 teaspoon sweet paprika
Salt and freshly ground black pepper to taste
   In a large glass bowl, combine the barley, green and red sweet peppers, and corn. In a small glass bowl, whisk together vinegar, olive oil, basil,

parsley, paprika, salt, and pepper. Pour vinegar mixture over the barley mixture and toss until all ingredients are coated. Cover and refrigerate for several hours before serving to allow flavors to blend.

Side dishes

PICKLED BEETS
1 can sliced beets
1 medium-sized onion, very thinly sliced
2 cloves garlic, halved
1/3 cup red wine
1/3 cup vinegar
1 tablespoon honey
1/4 teaspoon salt
6 peppercorns
4 whole cloves
1 bay leaf
1 teaspoon celery seed

Drain beets, reserving 3/4 cup liquid. Arrange beets alternately with onion slices in quart jar; add garlic. In saucepan combine reserved 3/4 cup beet liquid with all remaining ingredients; bring to boil; pour over contents of jar. Let stand uncovered at room temperature until cold, then cover and chill at least 24 hours before serving. It's a good idea to shake the jar gently now and then so that seasonings will be evenly distributed.

SPICED PICKLED EGGS
12 small eggs, hard-cooked and peeled
1 small onions, thinly sliced

3 cups vinegar
One 3-inch cinnamon stick
1 tablespoon honey
1 teaspoon whole allspice
1 teaspoon whole cloves
1/2 teaspoon whole coriander seeds
1 quarter-size slice fresh ginger
1 bayleaf
Place eggs and onion in a wide-mouth jar. Combine remaining ingredients in a nonreactive saucepan over medium heat. Bring the mixture to a boil, reduce the heat to low, and simmer for 5 minutes. Pour over the eggs. Cover and refrigerate for a week before serving. Eggs will keep about two months in the refrigerator.

STUFFED PEPPERS

Stuff large green peppers with cabbage slaw and stack in a stone crock. Cover with vinegar and age 4 weeks before using.

SPICED MUSHROOMS

1 pound fresh mushrooms
1/2 cup vinegar
1 teaspoon soy sauce
1 teaspoon hot pepper sauce
1 tablespoon olive oil
1 tablespoon ginger
3 cloves garlic, peeled and chopped
Blanch mushrooms in boiling water for 2 minutes, drain and pat dry. Put all ingredients into a jar with a tight lid and refrigerate overnight. Pile

these mushrooms on spinach leaves and serve with hot garlic toast.

GLAZED RED ONIONS
2 tablespoons olive oil
1 large red onion, thinly sliced
1 tablespoon raisins
3 tablespoons vinegar
2 teaspoons fresh thyme, minced
1/2 teaspoon honey
Salt and freshly ground black pepper to taste
Warm oil in a heavy nonreactive skillet over medium heat. Add onion and sauté, stirring often, until softened, or about 5 minutes. Add remaining ingredients and stir well. Cook until glaze is thickened, or about 4 minutes. Season with salt and pepper. Serve warm or at room temperature.

ZUCCHINI WITH SOUR CREAM AND THYME
3 tablespoons olive oil
1 pound zucchini, shredded
2 tablespoons vinegar
2 teaspoons fresh thyme, minced
1/2 cup nonfat sour cream
Salt and freshly ground black pepper to taste
In a heavy nonreactive skillet, warm oil over medium heat. Add the squash and sauté until golden, or about 4 minutes. Remove and set aside. Add the vinegar to the pan, scraping up any bits at the bottom. Cook until reduced to a teaspoon. Add thyme and sour cream, mixing well. Return squash to skillet and stir to coat. Heat through and season with salt and pepper.

DILLED POTATOES
1/4 cup canola or olive oil
1 pound small red new potatoes, cut in half
3 tablespoons vinegar
3 tablespoons fresh dill, minced
Salt and freshly ground black pepper to taste

In a heavy nonreactive skillet, warm the oil over medium heat. Add the potatoes and sauté, stirring frequently, until lightly browned and tender, or about 15 minutes. Add vinegar and cook for another 3 minutes. Sprinkle with dill and season with salt and pepper.

CARROTS AND FENNEL
2 tablespoons butter
1/2 cup onion, finely chopped
1 clove garlic, minced
2 cups carrots, peeled and thinly sliced
1/2 cup tomato, peeled, seeded, and diced
3 tablespoons vinegar
3 tablespoons fresh fennel, minced
2 tablespoons water
Salt and pepper to taste

In a nonreactive saucepan, melt butter over medium heat. Add onion and garlic. Stirring, sauté until translucent, or about 3 minutes. Add carrots, tomato, vinegar, fennel, and water. Cover, reduce heat to low, and simmer just until carrots are tender, or about 6 to 10 minutes. Season with salt and pepper.

CABBAGE AND JALAPENO SLAW
4 cups cabbage, finely shredded
1 1/2 cups sweet red pepper, cored, seeded, and diced
1/2 cup green onion, thinly sliced
1 fresh jalapeno pepper, cored, seeded, and minced
1 clove garlic, minced
1 tablespoon fresh marjoram, minced
1/4 cup olive oil
1/4 cup vinegar
1 tablespoon water or dry white wine
1/2 teaspoon ground cumin seeds
1/2 teaspoon honey
Salt and pepper to taste

    In a large nonreactive bowl, toss together cabbage, red pepper, green onion, jalapeno pepper, garlic, and marjoram. In small nonreactive bowl, whisk olive oil, vinegar, water or wine, cumin, sugar, salt, and pepper. Pour dressing over slaw. Toss lightly to mix well. Cover; refrigerate several hours.

SWEET-AND-SOUR LENTILS
2 cups vegetable stock or water
1 cup dry lentils
2 tablespoons canola or olive oil
1/2 cup onion, chopped
1 clove garlic, minced
1 jalapeno pepper, cored, seeded, and minced
1/4 cup vinegar
2 tablespoons honey
1/4 teaspoon ground cloves

1 tablespoon fresh parsley, minced

 Combine stock or water and lentils in a heavy saucepan and bring to a boil over medium-high heat. Reduce heat to low, cover saucepan, and cook until tender, or about 25 minutes. In a large, heavy nonreactive skillet, warm oil over medium heat. Add onion, garlic, and jalapeno pepper and sauté until softened, or about 5 minutes, stirring occasionally. Stir in vinegar, honey, and cloves and cook for 1 minute. Stir in cooked lentils and parsley.

BAKED BEANS
1/2 pound dry pinto beans
2 tablespoons canola or olive oil
1 cup onion, chopped
2 cloves garlic, minced
1 tablespoon fresh ginger, minced
1 jalapeno pepper, cored, seeded, and minced
1 1/2 cups apple cider
1/2 cup vinegar
2 tablespoons molasses
2 tablespoons packed light brown sugar
1 tablespoon Dijon mustard
1 bay leaf
1 tablespoon fresh thyme, minced
Salt and freshly ground black pepper to taste

 Rinse beans, place in a large bowl, and cover with cold water. Let sit overnight, or at least 8 hours. Drain and put into a nonreactive ovenproof casserole. Preheat oven to 350 degrees. In a heavy nonreactive skillet, warm the oil over medium heat. Add the onion, garlic, and jalapeno pepper. Sauté until softened, or about 5 minutes, stirring occasionally. Stir into the beans with the remaining ingredients. Cover and bake until beans are tender, or about 2 to 3 hours.

Meats

BARBECUED CHICKEN BREASTS

8 green onions, chopped
1/4 cup garlic red wine vinegar
2 tablespoons canola or olive oil
1 tablespoon soy sauce
2 teaspoons ground allspice
1 fresh green jalapeno cored and seeded
1/2 teaspoon freshly ground black pepper
1/2 teaspoon ground cinnamon
1/4 teaspoon ground nutmeg

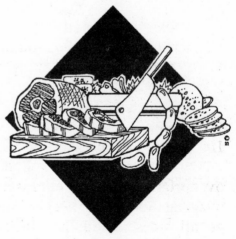

4 skinless, boneless chicken breast halves
Combine onions, vinegar, oil, soy sauce, allspice, hot pepper, black pepper, cinnamon, and nutmeg in a blender or food processor and puree. Pour puree into a shallow nonreactive dish. Add chicken breasts, turning to coat. Cover and refrigerate 4 hours, turning occasionally. Remove chicken from marinade and grill over medium-hot coals until

cooked through, or about 20 minutes, turning several times.

BEEF STEW WITH HERBS
2 tablespoons canola or olive oil
1 1/2 pounds beef chuck, cut into 1-inch pieces
1/2 cup vinegar
1/3 cup tomato sauce
3 medium tomatoes, peeled, seeded, and chopped
1 tablespoon honey
1 teaspoon salt
2 cloves garlic, minced
1 teaspoon fresh rosemary, minced
1/2 teaspoon ground cinnamon
1/2 teaspoon ground cumin seeds
1/2 teaspoon freshly ground black pepper
1/4 teaspoon ground cloves
1 bay leaf
1 cup water
1 1/2 pounds pearl onions, peeled
1/4 cup fresh parsley, minced

Preheat oven to 300 degrees. In a heavy ovenproof nonreactive casserole pan, warm the oil over medium-high heat. Add the beef and brown on all sides. Add the vinegar, tomato sauce, tomatoes, honey, salt, garlic, rosemary, cinnamon, cumin, black pepper, cloves, and bay leaf and stir. Add the water, onions, and parsley. Cover and bring to a boil, then place in oven. Bake for 1 hour, or until the meat is tender, adding water if necessary. Remove bay leaf before serving.

LAMB STEW WITH FENNEL SAUCE

2 pounds lean, boneless lamb, cut into 1-inch squares
2 tablespoons canola or olive oil
2 cups beef or vegetable stock, or water, boiling
1 cup vinegar
3 tablespoons fresh fennel, minced
1 teaspoon salt
1/2 teaspoon freshly ground black pepper
2 tablespoons butter
2 tablespoons whole wheat flour
2 cups beef or vegetable stock
1 1/2 tablespoons vinegar
1 large egg yolk, beaten until lemon-colored

Heat oil in a large, heavy nonreactive pan over medium heat. Add lamb cubes and cook until browned on all sides. Add boiling stock or water, vinegar, 1 tablespoon fennel, salt, and pepper. Bring to a boil, reduce heat to low, cover, and simmer for about 1 hour, or until tender.

About 15 minutes before the lamb is done, prepare the sauce. In a heavy, nonreactive saucepan, melt butter over medium heat and stir in flour until smooth. Add stock gradually, stirring constantly to keep the mixture smooth. Reduce heat and cook for 10 minutes, stirring occasionally. Remove from heat and stir in remaining fennel, vinegar, and egg yolk. When lamb is tender, drain and place on a platter and serve with sauce and whole wheat noodles or boiled new potatoes.

Chapter 8

HOW THESE SUPERFOODS HEAL

You know you are getting older when all the names in your little black book end in "M.D.". Robert Orben, comedian.

❀ PERSONAL PROFILE. KW was the picture of health and radiance--at age 89. She walked and talked like a healthy 40 year old woman, with no limitations. I met her at a health trade show where she was helping a friend with an exhibit booth. When I asked KW what her secret was for halting the processes of time, she replied: "Nutrition!!". Since a child, KW had been reared on simple farm cooking, where her parents had little money for the expensive sweets that people in the city buy. When she got married, she became more interested in nutrition and read some books that gave her more insight. She had outlasted two husbands, had her original teeth, an infectious smile, and more energy than most teenagers. Among the secrets she shared with me were her customs of regularly eating garlic, honey, and vinegar. She also used vinegar as a shampoo rinse and used a honey and oatmeal face pack recipe that is found in the honey recipe chapter. While many Americans dread the prospects of old age and the compromises in function, KW was proof that you can definitely slow down the aging process if you are willing to commit some time and energy to wellness. We either make time for wellness, or we will be forced to make time for illness.

Wouldn't it be nice if the answers were so simple? If instead of struggling through a maze of pain, suffering, doctors, hospitals, surgeries, and drugs; a person could find relief in simple and inexpensive healers from Nature? If instead of spending trillions of dollars on ineffective therapies and billions of dollars on high tech research, we could prevent the common nasty diseases in America with some good old fashion home remedies. Good news!! The answers to your health problems can be quite simple and elegantly effective!!

In this book, you have visited with some of Nature's wondrous healing agents: honey, garlic, and vinegar. Now that you have read this far, you might be interested in finding out why nutrition, in general, and specifically these three superfoods can be so helpful in supercharging your health.

> ## The main points of this chapter are:
> 1) All creatures on earth rely heavily of the quality and quantity of nutrient intake for their health and longevity.
>
> 2) We are facing a serious "health care meltdown" in which our huge investment in a "drugs and surgery" has not rescued us from sickness and early death. We cannot buy health, we must earn it through a healthy lifestyle, including these superfoods.
>
> 3) The majority of Americans are malnourished due to poor choices at the dinner table. Our quantity of food intake is enough, and maybe too much. But our quality of choices is way off. We eat too much of the wrong stuff and not enough of the right stuff.
>
> 4) The body wants to be well. By nourishing the "life forces" within, you set the stage for wondrous miracles of health to occur. Nutrition, exercise, attitude, detoxification, body maintenance, and genetics are the greatest forces that influence our health.

THE IMPORTANCE OF NUTRITION

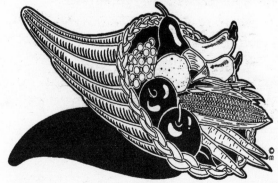

Nutrition and health. It makes so much sense: "you are what you eat." Veterinarians know the irreplacable link between nutrient intake and health. Actually, most of our pets eat better than most Americans. Your dog or cat probably eats a balanced formula of protein, carbohydrate, fat, fiber, vitamins and minerals. Yet, most humans choose our foods based upon taste, cost, emotional needs and convenience. The most commonly eaten food in America is heavily refined and nutritionally bankrupt white flour. Meanwhile, our livestock eat the more nutritious wheat germ and bran that we discard from whole wheat.

When our crops are not doing well, we examine the soil for nutrients, fluid and pH content. Our gardens prosper when we water, fertilize, and add a little broad spectrum mineral supplement. A sign posted near the junk food vending machines in a major city zoo warns: "Do not feed this food to the animals or they may get sick and die." Think about it. Do you think that the food that might kill a 400 pound ape is okay for a 40 pound child who is biologically very similar? If our gardens, field crops, pets, exotic zoo creatures and every other form of life on earth are all heavily dependent on their diet for health, then what makes us think that humans have transcended this dependence?

As Americans have compiled among the world's highest incidences of heart disease, cancer, stroke, diabetes, arthritis, and obesity; we seem to ignore the irreplacable link between eating whole foods and good health. The Surgeon General of the United States reports that up to 65% of all disease could be prevented through proper nutrition.

There is a basic flaw in our thinking about health care in this country. We treat symptoms, not the underlying cause of the disease. Yet, the only way to provide long-lasting relief in any degenerative disease, like cancer, arthritis and heart disease, is to reverse the basic cause of the disease.

For example, let's say that the first thing I do every morning when I arrive at my office is to slam my thumb in the desk drawer. After the first few days, it really hurts. As I continue slamming my thumb each morning, the thumb turns black and blue. I go to the doctor for relief. Doctor A tells me: "I will give you a prescription for an anti-inflammatory agent, cortisone, to reduce the swelling in your thumb." I want another opinion. Doctor B tells me: "I will give you a prescription for an analgesic drug, to help you better tolerate the pain." I still am not convinced that I have the right answer, so I get a third opinion. Doctor C tells me: "I am going to have to amputate that thumb, since it is obviously defective." The real answer is "stop slamming your thumb in the desk drawer" or reverse the underlying problem and allow your natural healing forces to take over.

You might say that my little story has nothing to do with your health problem. Let's say that Mrs. Jones is suffering from degenerative rheumatoid arthritis. Her knuckles, hips, and other joints are so swollen that they limit Mrs. Jones's activities. In this case, she could reverse the disease by avoiding the allergenic foods of dairy and wheat, while also taking supplements of fish oil, zinc, pantothenic acid, and bee pollen. Doctor A tells her: "I will give you a prescription for an anti-inflammatory agent, cortisone, to reduce the swelling in your joints." Doctor B tells her: "I will give you a prescription for an analgesic drug, to help you better tolerate the pain." Doctor C tells her: "I am going to have to do hip replacement surgery because those joints are defective." The correct answer is to change the underlying causes of the disease, or "stop slamming your thumb in the drawer".

In the American health care system, we usually shift symptoms with medication or surgery, as if in a bizarre "shell game", when we really need to deal with the fundamental cause of the disease. Nutrition, and in particular, the superfoods highlighted in this book will help change the underlying cause of many health problems.

Another example is heart disease. There are over 60,000 miles of blood vessels in the average adult body. When a person develops blockage in the arteries near the heart, open heart bypass surgery will be recommended for 360,000 Americans this year. In this procedure, a short section of vein from the leg is used to replace the plugged up vessels near the heart. But what has been done to improve the other 59,999 miles left that are probably equally obstructed? A Harvard professor, Dr. E. Braunwald, investigated the records from thousands of bypass patients in the Veteran's Administration Hospitals and found no improvement in lifespan after this expensive and risky surgery.[1] Why? Because the underlying cause; which could be a complex array of diet, exercise, stress, and toxins; has not been resolved. Bypass surgery treats the symptoms of heart disease like chemo and radiation treat the symptoms of cancer. Each provide temporary relief, but no long term cure.

Meanwhile, Dr. Dean Ornish has spent years developing a program that could reverse heart disease, something that drugs and surgery cannot do. His program recently was found effective in a clinical study. When you deal with the underlying causes of a degenerative disease, you are more likely to get long term favorable benefits. When you allow the cause of the disease to continue and merely treat the symptoms, then the disease just keeps getting worse. In hundreds of diseases and billions of patients, this obvious law holds true.

LEARNING NUTRITION FROM NATURE

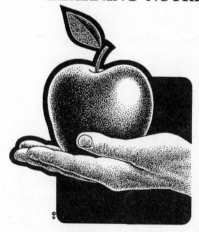

Without food processing we wouldn't know much about human nutrition. That's right. When European sailors spent months at sea with an imbalanced diet lacking in fresh fruits and vegetables, they came down with scurvy. Half of all trans-oceanic explorers from 1600-1850 died from this common vitamin C deficiency. When we taught the Indonesians how to refine whole rice down to white rice, thus removing the valuable thiamin, we began the beri-beri (literally means "I cannot, I cannot") disease of thiamin deficiency. When we decided to remove the fiber from whole fruits, vegetables and grains, we began history's greatest epidemic outbreaks of obesity, heart disease, cancer

and more. When we naively thought that we could
duplicate the nutritional value of mother's milk for
newborn infants, we later learned of all the minute
but critical components in mother's milk.

Everytime we think that we can improve on
nature, we find our confidence misplaced.
Everytime we fiddle with a wholesome food, we
erode its nutrient value. In whole foods lies a
universe of nutrients that we will never fully
understand but are there for our benefit.
Extracting juice from fruits and vegetables makes
as much sense as eating white flour.

Nature has spent billions of years fine tuning
our nutrient intake. Food is a rich tapestry of
thousands of substances. Food contains life-giving
agents that we are only beginning to understand.
One third of all prescription drugs in America
originated as plant products. It is food that
provides macronutrients, like carbohydrate, fat and
protein, that drive extremely influential hormones
and prostaglandins in your body. It is food that
establishes your pH balance and electrolyte "soup"
that bathes every cell in your body. It is food that
contains all the vitamins, minerals, and "sub-
nutrients" that have become a hotly researched
area. While vitamin and mineral supplements are
valuable, they cannot replace the fundamental
importance of a wholesome diet.

Our eating habits are all acquired. We base
our current diet on what mother cooked when we
were younger; what our society, ethnic and
religious groups prefer; what is advertised in print
and electronic media, and what is available in the

local grocery store. People in the Phillipines or the Amazon are born with structurally identical taste buds to Americans, yet they eat entirely different foods. Realize that it takes about 3 weeks to acquire new eating habits. Try the recipes in this book for 3 weeks, at which time it will become easier to stay with this new found way of eating; and you will probably find that the nutrient-depleted junk food of yesterday really doesn't satisfy your taste buds like whole foods.

SYNERGISTIC FORCES IN WHOLE FOODS

Although 1000 mg daily of vitamin C has been shown to reduce the risk for stomach cancer, a small glass of orange juice containing only 37 mg of vitamin C is twice as likely to lower the chances for stomach cancer. Something in whole oranges is even more chemo-protective than vitamin C. Although most people only absorb 20-50% of their ingested calcium, the remaining calcium binds up potentially damaging fats in the intestines to provide protection against colon cancer.

In 1963, a major "player" in the American drug business, Merck, tried to patent a single antibiotic substance that was originally isolated from yogurt. But this substance did not work alone. Since then, researchers have found no less than 7 natural antibiotics that all contribute to yogurt's unique ability to protect the body from infections. There are many anti-cancer agents in plant food, including beta-carotene, chlorophyll, over 800 mixed carotenoids, over 20,000 various bioflavonoids, lutein, lycopenes and canthaxanthin.

The point is: we can isolate and concentrate certain factors in foods for use as therapeutic supplements, but we must always rely heavily on the mysterious and elegant symphony of ingredients found in whole food, especially the superfoods of garlic, honey, and vinegar.

DIETARY RECOMMENDATIONS

Since the 1964 World Health Organization published their first pamphlet on cancer causes, many prominent health organizations have publicized their own personal version of a "healthy diet". Guidelines on good eating principles have come from the Senate Diet Goals, American Cancer Society, American Dietetic Association, Surgeon General of the United States, United States Public Health Association, American Heart Association, and many more. While these programs have minor variations, they have much in common. Each of these programs embraces a diet that:

-uses only unprocessed foods, nothing in a package with a label

-uses high amounts of fresh vegetables

-employs a low fat diet

-emphasizes the importance of regularity

-uses low fat dairy or no dairy products, with yogurt as the preferred dairy selection

-stabilizes blood sugar levels with no sweets and never eat something sweet by itself

-increases potassium and reduces sodium intake

OUR CURRENT HEALTH CARE "MELTDOWN"

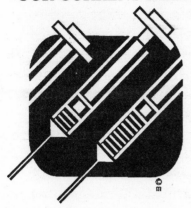

America spends over $1 trillion each year on what we call "health care", which is more "disease maintenance" than anything else. America is number 1 in the world for health care expenses, but number 27 among countries for lifespan. We spend twice the money per capita compared to any other nation on earth for health care. And our "health state of the union" is less than spectacular:

-58 million Americans have high blood pressure
-half of us die from heart disease and one fourth from cancer, both diseases were relatively unknown until this century
-24 million have insomnia
-50 million have regular headaches
-55 billion aspirin consumed yearly
-9 million alcoholics
-40% are overweight
-40 million have mental illness
-9.6 million older adults each year suffer drug-induced side effects, including 659,000 hospitalizations and 163,000 with memory loss
-we have a worse infant survival record than such undeveloped countries as Venezuela and the Phillipines.

Apparently, we cannot buy good health, but must earn it through nourishing the natural healing forces within our bodies. This nourishing process begins with good nutrition, with the pivotal superfoods of vinegar, garlic, and honey.

When the doctor sets a broken bone, he or she does not heal the patient, but rather sets in place the tissue so that Nature can heal us from within. Same thing happens in stitching up a cut, or when you recovered from your last bought with the flu. The only way you stay well or heal from a health challenge is by nourishing that "life force" within us. When we stop trying to repeal the laws of Nature and start cooperating within the framework of non-negotiable natural biochemical laws, then we will find a quantum leap in our health and improved results at the doctor's office.

USE AND ABUSE OF MODERN MEDICINE

Think of a sink overflowing with a mess of water all over the floor. Our medical system spends an incredible amount of time and money trying to wipe up the mess on the floor when the easiest solution is to turn off the faucet. Dr. Christiaan Barnard, the pioneering heart transplant surgeon, claims that the greatest progress in health care in the last 500 years came from, not a drug or surgical procedure, but the invention of the indoor flushing toilet, thus eliminating the many plagues caused by contaminated water supplies.

Throughout most of the world and recorded history, natural healing agents were the main tools of the physician, with herbs serving as the favored medicines. Avicenna was an Arab herbalist who lived in the 11th century and travelled extensively throughout the known world to catalog the medical uses of herbs. He eventually wrote 100 books on this subject, culminating in his 1 million word tome: CANON OF MEDICINE. This book was considered a standard for medical education throughout Europe and Asia until the 17th century. Garlic, vinegar, and honey were mentioned throughout this textbook.

The big shift in medical outlook began with a Swiss physician, Theophrastus von Hohenheim, who became discontent in the early 16th century with his training and began wandering Europe. While in the mines in Italy, Hohenheim was intrigued by the refining of minerals. He took this knowledge and began using mercury to treat his patients. He further dabbled in the use of strong minerals for medicines. His methods were widely criticized and he died after being tossed from a window by his adversaries while only 50 years old.

Around 1850, a French chemist, Louis Pasteur, found that heat could kill the tiny organisms that caused infections. Pasteur also worked on weakening the bacteria and injecting them into healthy people to prevent the disease--a process we now accept widely as vaccination. In 1910, Abraham Flexner wrote his famous report, MEDICAL EDUCATION IN THE UNITED STATES AND CANADA, which highly criticized all forms of healing except allopathy, which uses strong drugs to treat conditions. Practitioners of herbal or naturopathic medicine were ushered out of town, and the era of monopoly control by drug and surgery-oriented medical doctors began.

By 1928, Alexander Fleming had taken penicillin from bread mold and injected it into a patient with an infection. The recovery process was astoundingly quick and the era of anti-biotics was born. By the end of World War II, the development of chemicals were coming faster than they could be cataloged or tested for safety. The chemical age was born, and with it came the mixed blessings of miracle materials and the immoral contamination of our lovely planet. In the 1950s, Jonas Salk brought us the polio vacccine, and helped to end one of the worst scourges of mankind.

There is a difference between using our knowledge to improve our lot and abusing our knowledge through ego to worsen our lot. Drugs and surgery have their places in the healing arts, especially as short term fixes to get an acutely ill patient through a crisis phase. There are times when no other form of healing will work. But when we rely on these invasive therapies to heal a problem which can only be healed by encouragin our natural healing processes, then we end up worse off. We need to be more restrained with medical therapies and more liberal with natural healing therapies. The intelligent combination would leave us with astoundingly good health.

Many sick people are defying all of Nature's laws: poor diet, smoking, no exercise, too much stress, no quiet time, and a body loaded with toxins. Without a thought for changing this semi-suicidal lifestyle, the doctor will put the patient on an endless array of prescription drugs, which all have dastardly side effects, until the patient eventually develops a really serious disease, like cancer. We arrogantly assume that drugs can reverse the abuse caused by decades of poor nutrition and toxic burden. We are not respecting the laws of nature. Oftentimes, the answers to complex modern health problems are as simple as bringing in the Dream Team of superfoods.

MALNUTRITION IN AMERICA--THE GREAT NUTRITION ROBBERY
"I saw a few die of hunger, but of overeating a hundred thousand." Benjamin Franklin

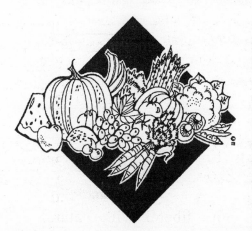

Howard Hughes, the multi-billionaire, died of malnutrition. It is hard to believe that there can be malnutrition in this agriculturally abundant nation of ours--but there is. At the time of the Revolutionary War, 96% of Americans farmed while only 4% worked at other trades. Tractors and harvesting combines became part of an agricultural revolution that allowed the 2% of Americans who now farm to feed the rest of us. We grow enough food in this country (quantity) to feed ourselves, to make half of us overweight, to throw away enough food to feed 50 million people daily, to ship food overseas as a major export, and to store enough food in government surplus bins to feed Americans for a year if all farmers quit today. With so much food available, how can Americans be malnourished?

The answer is: poor food choices along with major nutrient robbery. Americans chose their food based upon taste, cost, convenience and psychological gratification--thus ignoring the main reason that we eat, which is to provide our body cells with the raw materials to grow, repair and fuel our bodies. We take basically nutritious foods and take out good stuff, add bad stuff, and increase the cost substantially. The nutrients were in that food for a very good reason. The most commonly eaten foods in America are white bread, coffee and hot dogs. Based upon our food abundance, Americans could be the best nourished nation on record. But we are far from it.

We take Nature's elegantly designed
nutritious foods and:
•use drugs, hormones, and antibiotics to raise
animals faster, while spraying 1.2 billion pounds of
pesticides over our food crops
•fail to properly fertilize the soil with organic
matter and trace minerals and allow fields to lie
fallow, as was done throughout recorded history
•remove vitamins, minerals, and fiber during
extensive food processing
•add over 2800 Food and Drug
Administration approved additives, including salt,
fat, sugar, and unsafe food additives, like saccharin,
aspartame, and MSG
•dramatically increase the cost of the food,
which compounds the problems for the poor.

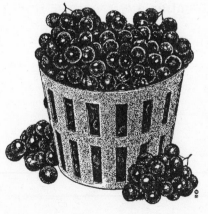

Over the course of millions of years of adaptation, the human body has developed a certain set of needs: whole food, exercise, rest, fresh air, sunshine, love. When we tamper with the extremely complex natural ingredients in our food supply, we usually wreak havoc on the food's nutritional content.

In the late 1930s, Dr. Weston Price, a dentist, and his wife, Monica, who was also a nurse, were intrigued by the possible link between diet and health.   In true "Indiana Jones" adventuresome fashion, they travelled the world logging over 100,000 miles on primitive aircraft to investigate 17 different cultures.   What they found was startling to scientists then: the more refined (read: adulterated) the food supply, the worse the health of the people.   Those people who ate their inherent diet had excellent health, teeth structure, energy, and appearance.   Those who deviated from their inherent diet suffered everything from mild symptoms, such as acne, skin and hair problems, and poor dental formation to the severest forms of mental retardation and even paralysis.

Another group of researchers in1988 from Emory University in Atlanta followed up on Dr. Price's work and found similar results.   They stated that the "paleolithic" hunter-gatherer diet of our ancestors was very different from our current refined diet, and that difference may contribute to many of our ailments.   Our ancestors ate a superior diet and enjoyed superior health, other than the frequent plagues from poor hygiene that would devastate entire regions.

> Overwhelming evidence from government surveys of 200,000 Americans and numerous respected universities shows that many Americans are low in their intake of:
>
> -VITAMINS: A, D, E, C, B-6, riboflavin, folacin, pantothenic acid
>
> -MINERALS: calcium, potassium, magnesium, zinc, iron, chromium, selenium; and possibly molybdenum and vanadium.
>
> -MACRONUTRIENTS: fiber, complex carbohydrates, plant protein, special fatty acids (EPA, GLA, ALA), clean water
>
> Meanwhile, we also eat alarmingly high amounts of: fat, salt, sugar, cholesterol, alcohol, caffeine, food additives and toxins.

This combination of too much of the wrong things along with not enough of the right things has created epidemic proportions of degenerative diseases in this country. The Surgeon General, Department of Health and Human Services, Center for Disease Control, National Academy of Sciences, American Medical Association, American Dietetic Assocation, and most other major public health agencies agree that diet is a major contributor to our most common health problems, including cancer and heart disease.

The typical American diet is high in fat while being low in fiber and vegetables. "Meat, potatoes, and gravy" is what many of my cancer patients lived on for decades. Data collected by the United

States Department of Agriculture from over 11,000
Americans showed that on any given day:

-41 percent did not eat any fruit

-82 percent did not eat cruciferous vegetables

-72 percent did not eat vitamin C-rich fruits
or vegetables

-80 percent did not eat vitamin A-rich fruits
or vegetables

-84 percent did not eat high fiber grain food,
like bread or cereal

The human body is incredibly resilient, which
sometimes works to our disadvantage. No one dies
on the first cigarette inhaled, or the first drunken
evening, or the first decade of unhealthy eating.
We misconstrue the fact that we survived this
ordeal to mean we can do it forever. Not so.
Malnutrition can be blatant, as the starving babies
in third world countries. Malnutrition can also be
much more slow and subtle; first bringing the
vague symptoms of chronic fatigue, constipation,
mood swings, poor wound recovery, and frequent
colds; followed by a decade of struggling with
incontinence, poor memory, pain in the chest, poor
digestion, and visual problems. Malnutrition in
America is a progressive and silent saboteur from
within the body, not an instant knockout punch.

It was the Framingham study done by
Harvard University that proclaimed: "Our way of
life is related to our way of death." While many
Americans are overfed, the majority are also poorly
nourished. The typical American, statistically
speaking, is overweight, has six colds per year, is
regularly plagued with lethargy, mild depression,

and constipation, gets dentures by age 45, begins a marked decline in function and vitality by age 50, and dies in their 60s or 70s from heart disease or cancer. Another scientist has stated the problem more bluntly: "We are digging our graves with our teeth."

YOUR BODY WANTS TO BE HEALTHY

"Nature alone cures, and what nursing has to do is put the patient in the best condition for Nature to act upon him." Florence Nightingale, founder of modern nursing, 1900

Once a folk medicine remedy can be explained, then it pole vaults into the higher ranking category of modern medicine. Most people don't need to understand how fire works in order to fully harness its energy. The same goes for the superfoods of vinegar, garlic, and honey; we don't need to fully understand how they help. We can capitalize on their amazing healing properties while scientists continue to better understand the healing properties of our food supply.

There is a growing list of folk medicine cures that have "graduated" to become modern medicine cures. Rauwolfia is an extract of the snakeroot plant, was used for centuries in the Far East for its tranquilizing effect. It is now prescribed by physicians to lower blood pressure. Reserpine, derived from rauwolfia, has been used by psychiatrists in treating severe mental disorders. For centuries foxglove was brewed by Indians to treat dropsy, which is a fluid accumulation in the legs caused by heart problems. Foxglove contributes the active ingredient, digitalis, which is now used as a prescription drug to stimulate weakened hearts. For centuries, a "poultice of bread mold" was applied to wounds to prevent infection. Penicillin was the active ingredient in bread mold. White willow bark contains aspirin and was used for centuries to treat aches and fevers, but was relegated to "folk medicine" status until a scientist received a Nobel prize for explaining how aspirin affects prostaglandins in the body.

My point in this lengthy discussion is quite simple. For centuries, garlic, honey, and vinegar have been mainstays in folk medicine to treat a wide assortment of ailments. The fact that we cannot fully explain how they work does not reduce their effectiveness. A substance does not stay in the folk medicine arsenal for centuries simply because of the "placebo effect", or belief in its action. Garlic, honey, and vinegar work. We can't always explain HOW they work, but their low cost, non-toxic track record, and wide availability should allow many readers to experience for themselves the healing power of these superfoods from Nature's pharmacy.

KNOW THE LAWS OF OPTIMAL NUTRITION
While the superfoods of garlic, vinegar, and honey should be consumed often, these foods do not represent a complete balanced diet. You need many other foods to create that complex puzzle that will keep you fit and energetic for the better part of a century. This section is designed to be a brief summary of the thousands of nutrition books available. You need to learn good judgment to chose the right foods to complement your superfoods of garlic, vinegar, and honey.

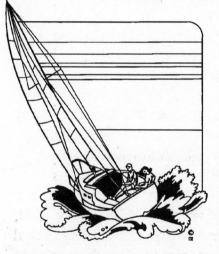

When sailing instructors teach you how to sail, they cannot show you around the world. They show you how to use the instruments of navigation-- a sextant, compass and map--and hope you can fare well on your own. So, too, I cannot follow you around for the rest of your life and make nutritional decisions for you. But I can condense the volumes of nutrition information into several easy-to-follow rules that become your navigation instruments in choosing the right foods. I have tried giving patients a detailed 2 week food intake program. By day 2, this patient is out of some food, then eats with a friend at a restaurant, then has dinner with the cousins--all of which throws the patient off their diet without any idea of knowing how to "wing it" or improvise. Use this section as a shortcut toward building good nutrition judgment in choosing foods and supplements that will prevent disease and build good health.

>The KISS (keep it simple, student) method of optimal nutrition.

-Go natural. Eat foods in as close to their natural state as possible. Refining food often adds questionable agents (like food additives, salt, sugar and fat), removes valuable nutrients (like vitamins, minerals, and fiber) and always raises the cost of the food. We are only beginning to fully appreciate the elegant symphony of nutrients available in whole foods. To naively and arrogantly believe that we can tamper with this time-tested formula and improve on it is just plain foolish. Therefore, shop the perimeter aisles of the grocery store, where you will find fresh vegetables and fruit, poultry, dairy, fish, meat, and bread. If you venture into the "deep dark interior" of the grocery store, then the quality of the food goes way down and the price goes way up.

-Expand your horizons. Eat a wide variety of foods. By not focusing on any particular food, you can obtain nutrients that may be essential but are poorly understood while also avoiding a buildup of any substance that could create food allergies or toxicities.

-Nibbling is better. Eat small frequent meals. Nibbling is better than gorging. Our ancestors

"grazed" throughout the day. Only with the advent
of the industrial age did we begin the punctual
eating of large meals. Nibbling helps to stabilize
blood sugar levels and minimize insulin rushes;
therefore has been linked to a lowered risk for
heart disease, diabetes, obesity and mood swings.

-Avoid problem foods. Minimize your intake
of unhealthy foods which are high in fat, salt, sugar,
cholesterol, caffeine, alcohol, processed lunch meats
and most additives.

-Seek out nutrient-dense foods. Maximize
your intake of life-giving foods, including fresh
vegetables, whole grains, legumes, fruit, low fat
meat (turkey, fish, chicken) and clean water. Low
fat dairy products, especially yogurt, can be
valuable if you do not have milk allergies or lactose
intolerance.

-Monitor your quality of weight, rather than
quantity of weight. Balance your calorie intake
with expenditure so that your percentage of body
fat is reasonable. Pinch the skinfold just above the
hipbone. If this skin is more than an inch in
thickness, then you may need to begin rational
efforts to lose weight. Obesity is a major factor in
cancer. Your quantity of weight is not nearly as
crucial as your quality of weight. Of all the
controversies the plague the nutrition field, one
issue that all nutritionists will agree on is to eat less
fat in your diet and store less fat in your body.

-Eat enough protein. Take in about 1 gram of
protein for each kilogram of body weight. Example:
150 pound patient. Divide 150 pounds by 2.2 to

find 68 kilograms, yields 68 grams of protein daily is needed to regenerate a healthy body.

-Use supplements in addition to, rather than instead of, good food. Get your nutrients with a fork and spoon. Do not place undo reliance on pills and powders to provide optimal nourishment. Supplements providing micronutrients (vitamins and minerals) cannot reverse the major influence of foods providing macronutrients (carbohydrate, fat, protein, fiber, water).

-If a food will not rot or sprout, then don't buy it or throw it out. Your body cells have similar biochemical needs to a bacteria or yeast cell. Foods that have a shelf life of a millenia are not going to nourish the body. Think about it: if bacteria is not interested in your food, then what makes you think that your body cells are interested? Foods that cannot begin (sprouting) or sustain (bacterial growth) life elsewhere, will have a similar effect in your body.

-Dishes should be easy to clean. Foods that are hard to digest or unhealthy will probably leave a mess on plates and pots. Dairy curd, such as fondue, is both difficult to clean and very difficult for your stomach to process. Same thing with fried, greasy or burned foods.

-Difference between surviving and thriving. Humans have survived car crashes at 200 miles per hour, falling out of jet planes without a parachute from five miles up, being fired out of cannons, inhumane treatment in prisoner of war camps, multiple gun shot wounds and a metal shaft fired cleanly through the head. While some people can survive a half century of smoking, no one thrives on it. Alcoholics can tolerate a suicidal lifestyle for decades. But their body and mind suffer and age rapidly in the process. None of these feats are good for the human body. Yet our tenacity is oftentimes our undoing. We assume that a diet that doesn't immediately kill us must be good for us. Not so.

Health and performance increase with increasing nutrient intake, until a plateau is reached. In pharmaceutical terms, there appears to be a "dose-dependent" response curve with the health benefits of many nutrients.

Think of the relative benefits of increasing daily intake of vitamin E:

-Most people can live on 10 international units (iu)

-Damage to the lungs from air pollution is reduced at 100 iu

-Heart disease is reduced at 200-400 iu

-Immune function is improved at 800 iu.

Humans can survive on 10 milligrams (mg) of vitamin C for decades. Yet, 90 mg lowers the incidence of ovarian cancer by 50%, while 300 mg increases lifespan in men by 6 years[2], and 10,000 mg helps to fight AIDS, cancer and the flu. Clearly, survival levels of nutrient intake are not enough for the person who wants to thrive.

-Nutrients as biological response modifiers (BRM). Know this rule: everything that you put in your mouth is a BRM. Brilliant scientists at the National Cancer Institute have labored for years trying to produce something from the laboratory that will rectify human cancer. These researchers have developed the field of BRM, in which potent drugs and extracts from the immune system will hopefully improve health. Results in this area have been very disappointing.

But everytime you eat a meal high in carbohydrates and get a little sleepy afterward, you have used food as a BRM to alter brain chemicals. A high salt diet changes the critical sodium to potassium ratio in the blood and cell membranes, which can affect many hormones and the permeability of cell membranes. Respect the incredible impact of food, water and air on the mind and body.

-The more wellness you have, the less illness you can have. Just like darkness is the absence of light, disease is the absence of wellness. Wellness is a state of optimal functioning of body, mind and spirit. A well person may have 90% wellness and 10% illness. A sick person may have 10% wellness and 90% illness. A body region cannot be well and ill at the same time. Therefore, curing illness is a matter of replacing it with wellness. The same unhealthy lifestyle may create heart disease in 30% of the people, cancer in 25%, arthritis in 10%, and mental illness in 5%. In a very important step toward removing illness, simply allow wellness to infiltrate the body and mind.

-Immune system--BOLSTERING THE BODY'S DEFENSE MECHANISMS. We have an extensive network of protective factors that circulate throughout our bodies to kill any bacteria, virus, yeast or cancer cells. Think of these 20 trillion immune cells as both your Department of Defense and your waste disposal company. It is the surveillance of an alert and capable immune system that defends most of us from infections, cancer, auto-immune diseases (like Multiple Sclerosis), allergies, and even premature aging.

In many people, for a variety of reasons, the immune system has not done its work.

The immune system can be _shut down_ by:
- -toxic metals, like lead, cadmium and mercury
- -volatile organic chemicals, from agriculture and industry
- -sugar
- -omega-6 fats, like soy and corn oil
- -stress and worry, and more.

The immune system can also be _enhanced_ by:
- -vitamins, like A, beta-carotene, C, E, and B-6
- -quasi-vitamins, like Coenzyme Q-10, EPA and GLA (special fats)
- -minerals, like zinc, chromium, and selenium
- -amino acids, like arginine and glutathione
- -herbal extracts, like echinecea, ginseng, Pau D'arco, and astragalus
- -nutrient factors, like yogurt, garlic, cabbage, enzymes and fresh green leafy vegetables.
- -positive emotions, like love, forgiveness and creative visualization

PARTING COMMENTS

✍ Congratulations for taking the time to read this far. Now you must put this knowledge into action. Buying an exercise device is a good start, but to gain any benefits you must use the device. Buying a book is a good start. Reading the book is a noteworthy accomplishment. But you must make a choice to incorporate these ideas into your lifestyle in order to gain any benefits. Promise to make one change in your health habits **today**. Make two changes tomorrow. Once you have gained some momentum, you will be surprised at how self-sustaining this lifestyle can be. May you live a long and fruitful life, full of zest, fulfilled dreams, and happiness.

---

[1]. Braunwald, E., New England Journal Medicine, vol.309, p.1181, Nov.10, 1983
[2]. Enstrom, J., Epidemiology, vol.3, p.194, May 1992

APPENDIX

📖

For more information

•Honey

Goodman, L. J., and Fisher, R. C., eds., The Behaviour and Physiology of Bees 1991 Gould, J. L. and C. G., The Honey Bee 1988

Hubbell, S., A Book of Bees 1988

Mech, D., Joy with Honey, 1994

Michener, C. D., et al., The Bee Genera of North and Central America 1994

Mitchell, J (ed), The Random House Encyclopedia, 1983

O'Toole, C., and Raw, A., Bees of the World 1992

Parkhill, J., The Wonderful World of Honey, 1993

Seeley, T. D., Honeybee Ecology 1985

Winston, M., The Biology of the Honeybee 1987

•Vinegar

Bragg, P, et al., Apple Cider Vinegar, 1985

Johnson, M. P., Gourmet Vinegars, 1990

Oster, M., Herbal Vinegar, 1994

Schmidt, R. M., Flavored Vinegars: Herb and Fruit 1988

Scott, C., Cider Vinegar,1973

Thacker, E., The Vinegar Book, 1995

•Garlic

Fulder, S., et al, Garlic, Nature's Original Remedy, 1991

Heinerman, J., The Healing Benefits of Garlic, 1994

Jensen, B., Garlic Healing Powers, 1992
Lau, B., Garlic for Health, 1988
Mindell, E., Garlic, the Miracle Nutrient, 1994
O'Brien, JE, The Miracle of Garlic & Vinegar, 1995

•Nutrition in General

Anderson, RA, Wellness Medicine, 1987
Carper, J., Food-Your Miracle Medicine, 1993
Carper, J., The Food Pharmacy, 1988
Colbin, A., Food and Healing, 1986
Haas, EM, Staying Healthy with Nutrition, 1992
Hausman, P., et al., Healing Foods, 1989
Hausman, P., The Right Dose, 1987
Hendler, SS, Doctor's Vitamin and Mineral
Encyclopedia, 1990
Jarvis, DC, Folk Medicine, 1958
Margen, S. (ed), The Wellness Encyclopedia of Food
and Nutrition, 1992
Murray, MT, et al., Encyclopedia of Natural
Medicine, 1990
Murray, MT, The Healing Power of Foods, 1993
Quillin, P., Beating Cancer with Nutrition, 1994
Quillin, P., Healing Nutrients, 1987
Salaman, M., Foods that Heal, 1989
Werbach, M., Nutritional Influences on Illness, 1993
Wood, R., Whole Foods Encyclopedia, 1988

NUTRITION PRODUCTS AVAILABLE BY MAIL ORDER

•Bulk Foods

Allergy Resources Inc., 195 Huntington Beach Dr., Colorado Springs, CO 80921, ph 719-488-3630

Deer Valley Farm, RD#1, Guilford, NY 13780, ph. 607-674-8556

Diamond K Enterprises, Jack Kranz, R.R. 1, Box 30, St. Charles, MN 55972, ph. 507-932-4308

Gravelly Ridge Farms, Star Route 16, Elk Creek, CA 95939, ph. 916-963-3216

Green Earth, 2545 Prairie St., Evanston, IL 60201, ph. 800-322-3662

Healthfoods Express, 181 Sylmar Clovis, CA 93612, ph. 209-252-8321

Jaffe Bros. Inc., PO Box 636, Valley Center, CA 92082, ph. 619-749-1133

Macrobiotic Wholesale Co., 799 Old Leicester Hwy, Asheville, NC 28806, ph. 704-252-1221

Moksha Natural Foods, 724 Palm Ave., Watsonville, CA, 95076, ph. 408-724-2009

Mountain Ark Co., 120 South East Ave., Fayetteville, AR, 72701, ph. 501-442-7191, or 800-643-8909

New American Food Co., PO Box 3206, Durham, NC 27705, ph. 919-682-9210

Timber Crest Farms, 4791 Dry Creek, Healdsburg, CA, 95448, ph. 707-433-8251, FAX -8255

Walnut Acres, Walnut Acres Road, Penns Creek, PA 17862, ph. 717-837-0601

•Mail Order Nutrition Companies
Bronson, 800-235-3200
Health Center for Better Living, 813-566-2611
NutriGuard, 800-433-2402
Terrace International, 800-824-2434
Vitamin Research Products, 800-877-2447
Vitamin Trader, 800-334-9310
Willner Chemists, 800-633-1106

•Stores that Sell Herbs by Mail
Blessed Herbs 800-489-HERB; fax 508-882-3755
Frontier Herbs 800-786-1388; fax 319-227-7966
Gaia Herbals, 800-994-9355
Herbal Healer Academy, 501-269-4177
San Francisco Herb Co. fax 800-227-5430
Star West 800-800-4372
Trout Lake Farm 509-395-2025

•Recommended Cookbooks 📖
American Cancer Society Cookbook, Anne Lindsay
American Health Food Book, Robert Barnett, Nao Hauser
Chez Eddy Living Heart Cookbook, Antonio Gotto Jr.
Eat Smart for a Healthy Heart Cookbook, Dr. Denton Cooley & Dr. Carolyn Moore
Eat Well, Live Well, Pamela Smith
Healthy Life-Style Cookbook, Weight Watchers
How to Use Natural Foods Deliciously, Barbara Bassett
Kathy Cooks Naturally, Kathy Hoshijo
Mix & Match Cooking for Health, Jennie Shapter
Natural Foods Cookbook, Mary Estella

Simply Light Cooking, Kitchens of Weight Watchers
Super Seafood, Tom Ney
The Healthy Gourmet Cookbook, Barbara Bassett
The I Can't Believe This has No Sugar Cookbook,
Deborah Buhr